T0213508

Broadly Engaged Team Science in Clinical and Translational Research

Debra Lerner • Marisha E. Palm
Thomas W. Concannon

Editors

Broadly Engaged Team Science in Clinical and Translational Research

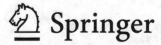 Springer

Editors
Debra Lerner
Tufts Medical Center
Boston, MA, USA

Marisha E. Palm
Tufts Medical Center
Boston, MA, USA

Thomas W. Concannon
RAND Corporation
Boston, MA, USA

ISBN 978-3-030-83030-4   ISBN 978-3-030-83028-1   (eBook)
https://doi.org/10.1007/978-3-030-83028-1

© Tufts Medical Center, RAND Corporation 2022
This work is subject to copyright. All rights are solely and exclusively licensed by the Publisher, whether the whole or part of the material is concerned, specifically the rights of translation, reprinting, reuse of illustrations, recitation, broadcasting, reproduction on microfilms or in any other physical way, and transmission or information storage and retrieval, electronic adaptation, computer software, or by similar or dissimilar methodology now known or hereafter developed.
The use of general descriptive names, registered names, trademarks, service marks, etc. in this publication does not imply, even in the absence of a specific statement, that such names are exempt from the relevant protective laws and regulations and therefore free for general use.
The publisher, the authors, and the editors are safe to assume that the advice and information in this book are believed to be true and accurate at the date of publication. Neither the publisher nor the authors or the editors give a warranty, expressed or implied, with respect to the material contained herein or for any errors or omissions that may have been made. The publisher remains neutral with regard to jurisdictional claims in published maps and institutional affiliations.

This Springer imprint is published by the registered company Springer Nature Switzerland AG
The registered company address is: Gewerbestrasse 11, 6330 Cham, Switzerland

Acknowledgments

The editors of this book would like to thank the following people for all of their hard work behind the scenes:

Grace Brown, Student Intern, Northeastern University

Nicholas Moustakas, MPhil, Research Development Specialist, Tufts Clinical and Translational Science Institute

Hannah Merrick Santos, MBA, Senior Project Manager, Tufts Clinical and Translational Science Institute

Kathy Siranosian, Consulting Editor, Corporate Writers, LLC

Nicole Tong, Research Project Coordinator, Tufts Clinical and Translational Science Institute

Amy West, MA, Manager of Communications and Media, Tufts Clinical and Translational Science Institute

This book was supported by the National Center for Advancing Translational Sciences, National Institutes of Health, Award Number UL1TR002544. The content is solely the responsibility of the authors and does not necessarily represent the official views of the NIH.

About the Book

Despite the large national investment in health science, and the vast and growing body of peer-reviewed research findings it has produced, a compelling body of evidence suggests that research too often has been slow, inefficient, and fallen short of desired impacts on health. Many are asking how research might be changed to be more innovative, less wasteful, and more responsive to unmet health needs. One emerging response within clinical and translational science, the motivation for this book, is to advance an approach that attempts to close the gap between research scientists and key stakeholders; the individuals and groups responsible for or affected by health-related decisions. Broadly engaged team science promises to support this aim by transforming the gold standard, multidisciplinary team science to include key stakeholders in activities across the research spectrum. These new roles and responsibilities range from generating research questions to implementing research projects, to aiding in the translation of discoveries from the laboratory to the community. A transition to broadly engaged team science reflects the idea that inclusivity and a diversity of perspectives are necessary to achieving progress in addressing complex health issues while representing a new benchmark for ethical research practice. This book is one of the first collections of papers describing how clinical and translational science researchers are defining and implementing new research practices and some of the successes and challenges involved. It represents the collective efforts of the Tufts Clinical and Translational Science Institute (CTSI) and its partner organizations. Tufts CTSI is supported by a grant from the National Center for Advancing Translational Science, within the National Institutes of Health. This book represents an initial and critical step toward organizing knowledge of broadly engaged team science and advancing the development of evidence-based practices. It includes examples of multidisciplinary, broadly engaged team science projects, the perspectives of academic leaders about the changes needed to encourage scientists to conduct broadly engaged team science, and a separate resource directory. Written in an accessible style, this book is intended to highlight the breadth of broadly engaged team science within the Tufts CTSI community, motivate researchers and stakeholders to build inclusive teams, bring rigor to often informal stakeholder engagement research practices, and encourage both practicing scientists and stakeholders to think more broadly about the development of scientific knowledge.

Contents

List of Figures

List of Tables

Chapter 1
Broadly Engaged Team Science at Tufts Clinical and Translational Science Institute

Alice M. Rushforth and Harry P. Selker

Abstract Tufts Clinical and Translational Science Institute (CTSI), from its start as a Clinical and Translational Science Award (CTSA) Program hub in 2008, has focused on practicing and promoting both multi-disciplinary team science and community-engaged research. This approach reflects the civic life and service focus of Tufts University and Tufts CTSI's inclusion of all schools across Tufts and multiple other academic and community organizations. It also reflects Tufts' strengths in community-based, health services, policy, and multidisciplinary team-based research. However, we found that implementing team science and community-engaged research as two distinct independent approaches failed to take advantage of potential synergies and left gaps in the translational continuum. To promote the synergies in these two approaches and to bridge gaps in optimal translation, we proposed a framework that merges these approaches and goes beyond involving stakeholders as advisors, to an approach that includes stakeholders as full team members, which we call "broadly engaged team science." This book reflects our journey in building and supporting broadly engaged team science by documenting current perspectives and practices and reflecting our continuing challenges to innovate and to foster widespread implementation.

Keywords Broadly engaged team science. · Science communication strategies. · Translational research.

Despite dramatic advances in biomedical science, translation into clinical care and impact on public health took far too long in the face of enormous need. Therefore, in 2006, the National Institutes of Health (NIH) launched the Clinical and Translational Science Award (CTSA) Program to move biomedical science discoveries more quickly and efficiently into practice and achieve real-world

A. M. Rushforth (✉)
Tufts Clinical and Translational Research Institute, Tufts Medical Center, Boston, MA, USA
e-mail: arushforth@tuftsmedicalcenter.org

H.P. Selker
Tufts Clinical and Translational Science Institute, Tufts University; Institute for Clinical Research and Health Policy Studies, Tufts Medical Center, Boston, MA, USA

© The Author(s), under exclusive license to Springer Nature Switzerland AG 2022

D. Lerner et al. (eds.), *Broadly Engaged Team Science in Clinical and Translational Research*, https://doi.org/10.1007/978-3-030-83028-1_1

benefits. Over the past 15 years, translational science has evolved significantly, with increased research funding, specialized journals and societies, and organizations across the world dedicated to this growing scientific discipline. To sharpen its focus on this work, in 2011, NIH established the National Center for Advancing Translational Sciences (NCATS), which took over the CTSA Program, "to transform the translational science process so that new treatments and cures for disease can be delivered to patients faster" [1]. Now, as the largest single program at NIH, over 60 CTSA hubs at academic health centers and universities provide research expertise, resources, services, education, training, and career development to investigators, all directed at accelerating translation into impact on health.

To fulfill the promise of having impact on health, the discipline of translational science was intended to be disruptive and to transform research practices with new and different approaches to research, education, and training. When introducing the CTSA Program, then NIH Director Elias Zerhouni identified "translational roadblocks" that needed to be surmounted in moving from the laboratory bench to the patient's bedside, and from demonstration at the bedside into clinical practice [2]. Soon, it was also noted that there were barriers further along the translational chain, to widespread and equitably distributed medical care, and to wide public benefit and policy. Focus on these translational roadblocks has been uppermost for CTSAs, including self-assessment in this mission and willingness to disrupt old approaches and to try new practices.

In carrying out this translational mission, CTSA hubs practice and promote both multi-disciplinary team science and community-engaged research, including a broad array of groups, organizations, and diverse individuals. Recognizing that academic institutions' structures and processes are legacies of infrastructure, policies, and practices built to support single-*discipline research,* in the 2014 CTSA Funding Opportunity Announcement (FOA), NIH tasked CTSAs with engaging their home institutions to update promotion and tenure policies to recognize and incentivize team science for all members of a translational team. At the same time, it was appreciated that, historically, community-engaged research has not been integrated into the path of research that starts at the bench and the research bedside. To address this, in the 2014 CTSA FOA, NIH also challenged CTSAs to take an experimental, data-driven approach to identify best practices for community engagement in all stages of research across the translational spectrum. This included addressing this need even in the early translational phases, which had not been common. Furthermore, based on the 2013 Institute of Medicine Recommendations Report on the CTSA Program, NIH also tasked CTSAs with embedding community engagement in "leadership, implementation, research, and communication strategies across all levels of the CTSA program" [3, 4].

Tufts Clinical and Translational Science Institute (CTSI), from its start as a CTSA hub in 2008, has focused on translation into impact on broadly practiced health care and health in the community. This approach reflects the civic life and service focus of Tufts University, Tufts Medical Center's pioneering role in advancing the science of patient-reported outcomes and health-related quality of life, and Tufts CTSI's inclusion of all schools across Tufts and multiple other academic and community organizations. It also reflects Tufts' strengths in community-based, health services, policy, and multidisciplinary team-based research.

In its early years, Tufts CTSI developed frameworks to identify stakeholders and guide engagement strategies, some described in later chapters of this book. We led development of the widely used 7Ps taxonomy for stakeholder engagement in research and the Six Stages of Comparative Effectiveness Research framework in 2012, and a systematic review of stakeholder engagement activities in Comparative Effectiveness Research in 2014 [5, 6]. To increase the research readiness of our communities, we collaborated with other Boston-area CTSAs and community organizations to publish a capacity-building primer for community engagement, *Building Your Capacity: Advancing Research through Community Engagement Curriculum Guide* [7, 8]. We also developed a new concept for partnered research, community-engaged pedagogy [9], provided innovative education and training to community members in a nationally recognized Community Fellows program, and sponsored efforts to build a coalition of community-based organizations in Boston's Chinatown, adjacent to the Tufts Health Sciences campus, through our Addressing Disparities in Asian Populations through Translational Research (ADAPT) initiative. ADAPT promotes sustained engagement to address historical tensions and mistrust in communities around research and investigators, with the long-term goal of shared action to address health concerns of greatest concern to the community [10, 11].

However, we found that implementing team science and community-engaged research as two distinct independent approaches failed to take advantage of potential synergies and left gaps in the translational continuum. To promote the synergies in these two approaches and to bridge gaps in optimal translation, we proposed a framework that merges these approaches and goes beyond involving stakeholders as advisors, to an approach that includes stakeholders as full team members, which we call "broadly engaged team science." To take full advantage of the potential contributions of diverse perspectives and experiences, broadly engaged team science holds that clinical and translational science must shift from using stakeholders as consultants, to *full membership of all stakeholders in the research team* [12].

This book reflects our journey in building and supporting broadly engaged team science by documenting current perspectives and practices and reflecting our continuing challenges to innovate and to foster widespread implementation. Broadly engaged team science is aligned with Tufts CTSI's vision and culture. Our identity as "The Extrovert CTSI" includes engaging a large number of diverse partners at the organizational and individual levels. We also include focusing on our collective impact by building multi-partner, multi-disciplinary, multi-stakeholder collaborations. However, putting theory into practice is challenging and we, like others, face acknowledged systemic roadblocks in an academic research culture deeply seated in single-disciplinary traditions.

Research has most relevance and impact when it addresses issues of importance to patients, communities, clinicians, caregivers, and others who make medical and health decisions. Additionally, to be optimally disseminated, which ultimately determines its impact, research must engage the healthcare system, industry, and policymakers. Incorporating these perspectives requires meaningful connections, collaboration, and full team membership of key stakeholders. Broadly engaged team science emphasizes that all relevant perspectives must be actively involved in posing research questions, defining meaningful outcomes, conducting research, interpreting findings, and disseminating results. This requires including the technical knowledge, skills, and the lived experience of diverse stakeholders. It also requires leadership that is committed to broad active inclusion in the joint work. As a research paradigm, this enhances study design and protocol development, the use of culturally sensitive study enrollment approaches, and the ultimate adoption of research results into practice. In turn, this provides the public with a greater return on its investment in research and promotes public engagement and trust in science. It also promotes development of an engaged, diverse research workforce.

We see this as being a natural progression. Historically, team science and community-engaged research developed as distinct research fields. However, both are grounded in similar foundational principles and values that we believe merge well into a larger unified approach as broadly engaged team science. Both fields are built on trust, respect, a shared vision among members of the research team, power-sharing and equity, melding of cultures, and flexibility and adaptability in pursuing goals. All varieties of both approaches involve purposeful team building, managing conflict, clear and timely communication, and setting clear expectations for roles, responsibilities, and acknowledgment. A byproduct of the distinct evolution of the team science and community-engaged research fields is that in each tradition different terms have often been used to describe similar activities. We hope this commonality will be evident throughout this book, even though we have not attempted to harmonize terms and concepts across approaches; rather we have honored the contexts and voices of contributing authors.

As we continue to try to put the concept of broadly engaged team science into authentic practice, and to promulgate broadly engaged team science practices across diverse departments, schools, and organizations, we are continually evolving our roadmap to a future where teams work seamlessly across fields, organizations, communities, and individuals. We examine our organizational structure and culture, the initiatives we support, and the services, education, and training we provide, all through the lens of broadly engaged team science. As we look to the future, there are many examples to draw inspiration from and areas in which we plan to develop further:

- The first and third sections of the book explore how broad engagement can transform research and improve treatments for patients. These demonstrate some of the ways in which the vision of broadly engaged team science is being realized at the organizational level and the team level. We are witnessing a transformation in the structure and culture of science leveraging new relationships and collaborative processes to improve impact on public health.

- In the second and fourth sections of the book, authors describe the principles and practices necessary for broadly engaged team science. At Tufts, we want to incorporate diverse stakeholders into CTSI governance, strategic management, and program planning. We are looking to do this by expanding our existing Stakeholder Expert Panel, which is comprised of representatives from diverse groups and citizens, to implement broadly engaged team science throughout all aspects of Tufts CTSI. As you will read, the goal is for diverse stakeholders to be an integral part of research management infrastructure as well as part of the research team.

- We, like many others, also recognize the need to find better ways to compensate and recognize stakeholders for the critical role they play on research teams. This includes, for faculty, adopting promotion and tenure criteria that acknowledge, reward, and incentivize broadly engaged team science. It also necessitates providing financial compensation to community stakeholders for the roles they perform on research teams.
- It is well-recognized that funding agencies and scientific journals have a role to play in promoting broadly engaged team science. While less in the purview of CTSAs and academic institutions, to the extent that we can in our advocacy and leadership roles, we will support needed changes in these key parts of the research enterprise to support broadly engaged team science to take hold at scale.
- We are developing and implementing new approaches to help investigators working at the earliest translational stages to identify and include relevant stakeholders in their research teams. Recognizing that different research projects will need to include stakeholders engaged in different activities and roles, a one-size fits all approach to broadly engaged team science does not work. Here a fit-for-purpose approach needs to be developed and deployed for each research team. In addition, frameworks and more general practical guidance and real-world examples on how to implement broadly engaged team science in basic and pre-clinical research are needed.
- We believe that broadly engaged team science should improve diversity, equity, and inclusion in research and thereby improve its impact on all of society. We recently completed an organizational anti-racism action plan that includes working with investigators to identify and involve relevant stakeholders in their work through a diversity, equity, and inclusion lens. We also will examine all Tufts CTSI programming, resources, services, training, and educational offerings to ensure the metrics for involvement of *diverse* stakeholders include race, ethnicity, socio-economic, and other considerations relevant to the social determinants of health.
- Throughout this book, authors stress the importance of developing, deploying, and providing training on science communication strategies that acknowledge community perspectives, find common ground, and engender a common purpose. The erosion of public faith in science jeopardizes clinical and translational research. To improve public understanding of the purposes and value of clinical research and to build and maintain trust among diverse participants, we are hosting dialogues on important scientific issues in communities with the goal of breaking down stereotypes, inspiring curiosity, building empathy, and enabling participants to link their health and well-being to their personal and civic

decision-making. We are also providing science communication training and education to researchers to enhance their ability to work in diverse, multi-discipline, multi-stakeholder research teams and to create a respectful team environment where all members can contribute as equals.

• Although broadly engaged research seeks to include diverse stakeholders as members of the research team, there are still challenges to its implementation. In addition to public mistrust in science and research that may limit engagement, for large sectors of society, public involvement in research may not be viewed as a civic or social responsibility. Also, it may not be perceived as linked to their own health and well-being or that of their community. Thus, we wonder if broadly engaged team science might be fostered by understanding cultural influences and applying practices that encourage and promote community volunteerism and civic engagement. How might we best expand knowledge and capacity for all members of society to be active agents in clinical and translational research? With clear examples of the impact of social movements on research, such as Act Up on AIDS research, promoting broadly engaged team science as civic engagement may help to increase public involvement in research and the impact of translational research on public health.

In summary, Tufts CTSI seeks to facilitate translational science across the full spectrum of translational biomedical and related research to achieve impact on health. We realize that this requires a broad commitment in our research and educational programs, organizational structures, and internal and external communications. Success will require engagement of institutional leaders and stakeholders and a comprehensive approach and plan. It also requires a focus on including all relevant disciplines and stakeholders. A major public undertaking that fails to include all relevant disciplines and partners, and only includes those in a single silo, would be incomplete and would reflect a limited and flawed vision. Why should we not have the same breadth of inclusion of disciplines, resources, perspectives, and capabilities in our academic enterprises that ultimately aim for real-world impact? We recognize that in academic institutions, there are challenges to these approaches, including, but not limited to, academic appointments, access to resources, financial accountability, and internal and external communications. Major efforts by institutional and university leadership are needed to become the cross-cutting academic and community-based enterprise that Tufts CTSI seeks to become, and we believe this will be worth the effort. Now, several years into this path, we believe that broadly engaged team science is an important approach for this work.

References

1. NIH National Center for Advancing Translational Sciences. https://ncats.nih.gov/ctsa/about. 2021
2. Zerhouni E (2005) Translational and clinical science - time for a new vision. N Engl J Med 335(15):1621–1623

3. Committee to Review the Clinical and Translational Science Awards Program at the National Center for Advancing Translational Sciences BoHSP, Institute of Medicine, Leshner, AI, Terry, SF, Schultz, AM, et al. (2013) The CTSA Program at NIH: Opportunities for Advancing Clinical and Translational Research. National Academies Press. https://www.ncbi.nlm.nih.gov/books/NBK144067/
4. Hudson KLR, Patrick-Lake B (2015) The precision medicine initiative cohort program – building a research foundation for 21st century medicine. Precision medicine initiative (PMI) working group report to the advisory committee to the director. NIH
5. Concannon TW, Meissner P, Grunbaum JA, McElwee N, Guise JM, Santa J, Conway PH, Daudelin D, Morrato EH, Leslie LK (2012) A new taxonomy for stakeholder engagement in patient-centered outcomes research. J Gen Intern Med 27(8):985–991. https://doi.org/10.1007/s11606-012-2037-1
6. Concannon TW, Fuster M, Saunders T, Patel K, Wong JB, Leslie LK, Lau J (2014) A systematic review of stakeholder engagement in comparative effectiveness and patient-centered outcomes research. J Gen Intern Med 29(12):1692–1701. https://doi.org/10.1007/s11606-014-2878-x
7. Leslie LR, Dawson E, Mulé C, Huang C, Pirie A, Mbawuike V, Rios M, Daudelin D, Allukian N (2012) Building your capacity: advancing research through community engagement
8. Hacker K, Tendulkar SA, Rideout C, Bhuiya N, Trinh-Shevrin C, Savage CP, Grullon M, Strelnick H, Leung C, DiGirolamo A (2012) Community capacity building and sustainability: outcomes of community-based participatory research. Prog Community Health Partnersh 6(3):349–360
9. Concannon TW, Fuster M, Saunders T, Patel K, Wong JB, Leslie LK, Lau J (2015) When and how are we engaging stakeholders in health care research? RAND Corporation
10. Rubin CL, Allukian N, Wang X, Ghosh S, Huang CC, Wang J, Brugge D, Wong JB, Mark S, Dong S, Koch-Weser S, Parsons SK, Leslie LK, Freund KM (2014) "we make the path by walking it": building an academic community partnership with Boston Chinatown. Prog Community Health Partnersh 8(3):353 363. https://doi.org/10.1353/cpr.2014.0046
11. Leclair A, Lim JJ, Rubin C (2018) Lessons learned from developing andsustaining a community-researchcollaborative through translational research. J Clin Translat Sci. Cambridge Univeristy Press 2(2):79–85. https://doi.org/10.1017/cts.2018.7
12. Selker HP, Wilkins CH (2017) From community engagement, to community-engaged research, to broadly engaged team science. J Clin Translat Sci. Cambridge Univeristy Press 1(1):5–6. https://doi.org/10.1017/cts.2017.1

Part I
Transforming Research with Broad Engagement

Chapter 2
The Transformative Power of Broadly Engaged Team Science: A Mother's Quest to Understand PXE

Sharon F. Terry

Abstract I came to the world of medical research not as a career choice, but as a response to an unexpected challenge, and my journey has been anything but typical. This chapter chronicles my quest to understand the disease pseudoxanthoma elasticum (PXE). I explain how adopting an open and collaborative approach led to not only the formation of PXE International, but also the establishment of the first clinical registry and biospecimen repository designed and managed by a lay advocacy disease organization and the discovery and patent of the gene associated with PXE. Today, PXE International's research collaborations have expanded worldwide as a natural history study, a biomarker study, and early trials in pyrophosphate (PPi) and other potential therapies commence. In addition, my recent work with the Genetic Alliance has led the way in putting people—individuals, families, and communities at the center of health research and services. We have contributed our leadership to help in the passage of the Genetic Information Nondiscrimination Act, the formation of the All of Us program, the establishment of the International Rare Disease Research Consortium, and many other international and national endeavors.

Keywords PXE international · pseudoxanthoma elasticum (PXE) · Patient Centered Outcomes Research Institute · PCORnet · Genetic Alliance

I came to the world of medical research not as a career choice, but as a response to an unexpected challenge, and my journey has been anything but typical. Once a college chaplain with a master's in theology, I never imagined that I would create the first clinical registry and biospecimen repository designed and managed by a lay advocacy disease organization or be the first and only lay person to discover and patent a gene discovery.

The journey began when, after a diagnostic odyssey, my two children were diagnosed with a rare genetic condition a few days before Christmas in 1994. They were

S. F. Terry (✉)
Genetic Alliance, Damascus, MD, USA
e-mail: sterry@geneticalliance.org

© The Author(s), under exclusive license to Springer Nature
Switzerland AG 2022
D. Lerner et al. (eds.), *Broadly Engaged Team Science in Clinical and
Translational Research*, https://doi.org/10.1007/978-3-030-83028-1_2

5 and 7 years old at the time. For several years, I had been in search of an answer as to why my daughter had a "rash" on her neck. The quest for their diagnosis came after my father and brother had both died terrible deaths that could have been handled better medically. Neither were consulted before undergoing major surgeries that would not prolong their lives. Two weeks before he died, my father had a colostomy for colon cancer with metastases to his liver and lungs. He felt shame about this and would have gladly forgone the surgery had he been given a clear picture of his extremely poor prognosis. My brother's doctors told him of a wonderful future that would be made possible by stereotactic radiosurgery for his glioblastoma multiforme. As we cajoled him to get out of bed and stop being lazy about his recovery, he was actually dying. A kind nurse told me that if he was her brother, she would cease treatment and prepare for his death, for his sake and for ours. His young wife, with their 10-month-old daughter, was not ready to hear that after being sold a different bill of goods. We rushed to get him what he needed to die.

I do not fault the teams of physicians in either case. I quickly discovered that we were not partners in the process of managing my loved ones' health; instead, we were expected to be the docile recipients of someone else's decisions. After the fact, it was clear to me that I should not accept any decision without evidence and discussion, and that I would have to be an advocate should anyone in my family face another medical dilemma. As a result, I did not accept that there was nothing wrong with my kids and doggedly pursued a diagnosis. And then, upon hearing the diagnosis of pseudoxanthoma elasticum (PXE), I went into overdrive to secure a position on the team that would determine what was or wasn't to be done.

The Formation of PXE International

Researching a disease was not easy in 1994, when the internet was rudimentary, and few people had access to online information. I had a master's in theology, with little background in any sort of science, let alone biology. To start, I copied and read hundreds of articles, most of which were case studies from medical journals. Though my understanding of methods, analysis, results, and thousands of complex and unfamiliar terms was sorely lacking, it seemed clear that these studies were not good representations of the PXE's characteristics or progression. Another enormous red flag to me were requests a day apart, from two different research groups, to take my children's blood to search for the disease's genetic marker. When I asked these two teams of scientists to share the samples, and not take blood from the kids twice, they scoffed at the idea and said they were in competition—a race to find the gene. As a parent, naïve to the process of scientific discovery, I was appalled.

All of this led my husband and me to establish PXE International. It appeared to us that the incentives of the research groups were not aligned with the individuals and families suffering from PXE. Fortunately, creating a nonprofit was not difficult in 1995, and there were many other support groups dedicated to helping people with diseases. A law firm in the Boston area, where we lived, incorporated the foundation and filed the 501 (c) (3) application for us, pro bono. Organizations like Genetic Alliance, an umbrella group that helped with starting and sustaining support groups, taught us the basics [1].

Collaborating with Patients Leads to the First Biospecimen Repository and Disease Registry Established by a Patient Advocacy Organization

The board of PXE International felt strongly that it was not enough to support people with the condition; they also wanted us to drive the research. Shortly after we had PXE International up and running, we began to search for other people with the condition. We quickly learned that most of those affected were adults in their 40s and 50s, often suffering with skin signs and vision loss, the major morbidities of the disease. I connected with many of these individuals by mailing pamphlets to ophthalmologists and dermatologists, and with their collaboration, PXE International became the first patient advocacy organization to establish a biospecimen repository.

We invited the affected individuals we located to donate blood to the PXE International BioBank. We also mailed an extensive 900-question survey to them, collecting information about their experience of living with PXE. We coded the responses to the paper survey and entered the data into a low cost, off-the-shelf software program, establishing the first disease registry with what is now called Patient Reported Outcomes (PROs). We also collected thousands of medical records— all paper, since this was before electronic health records existed—and blinded and scanned them to create a repository of information. Thus, we created our own real world evidence basis well before it was fashionable or encouraged. We did this in part to challenge a large cadre of researchers who felt that PROs would be useless information filled with bias from the person's lived experience. Once we had gathered PROs from 600 people, we analyzed information from 10 percent of them to determine how much concordance or discordance we saw compared to their medical record. We saw a great deal of concordance, and we also saw a good deal of misinformation in the medical records. We knew in 1996 that having both PROs and health records was critical if we were to understand the characteristics and progression of this condition.

Research Sparks Additional Collaborations, New Understanding, and Discovery of the PXE Gene

This information we gathered helped us discover several previously unknown aspects of PXE that I believe would not have been found without PROs. For example, women with PXE consistently reported that they were asked to have biopsies with every mammogram. Microcalcifications seen on the images had to be sampled to rule out cancer. As a result of these reports from women in our registry, we undertook a double-blind study, in which we examined the mammograms of 51 women with PXE and compared them to 109 controls. The mammograms of affected women all showed microcalcifications and none had cancer. Based on these results, we offered a new guideline to women and their clinicians: women with PXE have microcalcifications in the breast as a result of PXE, not as an indicator of a cancerous pathology [2]. We pursued a similar concern for men, precipitated by a urologist discovering testicular microlithiasis in a boy affected by PXE. This time we had to recruit participants, since imaging of the testes is not routine, and the discovery was analogous: men affected by PXE have testicular microlithiasis [3]. In both cases, the discoveries and resulting guidelines allayed a great deal of anxiety, unnecessary biopsies, and misinformation.

Early in our sojourn, we borrowed bench space at Harvard, and learned from post-docs late at night how to extract DNA, perform gel electrophoresis, score gels, and enter data in a spreadsheet. We shared our samples with our newly formed PXE International Research Consortium, with the requirement that they share with one another. In annual research meetings, we shared methods and results, and worked toward discovering the gene. In 1999, together with a number of research teams, we discovered that mutations in ABCC6, a membrane transport protein, were responsible for the autosomal recessive condition pseudoxanthoma elasticum (PXE). Along with a number of labs, we published the discovery, and then applied for a patent on the gene [4, 5]. We wanted to control the gene patent so that that we could freely share access to the gene and the variants found in it, rather than have a university technology transfer office gatekeep that access and/or create a proprietary database. PXE International licensed the gene for $100 in perpetuity to any labs that requested access. In turn, we required that the testing labs share all of the variants they found with PXE International. This prevented a proprietary database of mutations from being built since we published them online in the Leiden Open Variation Database (LOVD). These have since been transferred to ClinVar, where we verify and curate all of the variants we and others have found.

Expanding PXE International's Research Collaborations

Once we discovered the gene, we engaged a company looking to validate its technology to help us sequence the gene in hundreds of individuals around the world. We placed their instruments in Philadelphia, Honolulu, South Africa, and Belgium. I traveled, often with my kids whom I was homeschooling, to each of these areas, meeting with people affected by PXE in the regions around these labs and providing education, support, and asking for biological samples and PRO in exchange. PXE International brought these data together and explored whether there was a phenotype-genotype correlation, and though we did not discover one, we laid the groundwork for understanding the genetic basis of the disease. This, and extensive funding of labs in Budapest, Amsterdam, Modena, Cape Town, Hawaii, and eventually the founding of the PXE International Center of Excellence in Research and Clinical Care at Jefferson Medical College in Philadelphia, led to the discovery that ABCC6 facilitates the cellular efflux of ATP, which is rapidly converted into pyrophosphate (PPi), a major calcification inhibitor. This discovery has opened the door to many more research projects, closer to the translation end of biomedical research. In the past several years, PXE International's research collaborations have expanded to include several companies as a natural history study, a biomarker study, and early trials in PPi and other potential therapies commence.

Shortly after establishing the first biobank and registry run by a patient advocacy organization, with help from experts on human research ethics, biological specimen storage, and data science from the National Institutes of Health (NIH), the Centers for Disease Control and Prevention (CDC), and Genetic Alliance, many other patient advocacy organization founders and leaders came to ask me to help them establish biobanks and registries for their health conditions. With my children's permission, in 1996, I began to work with these other groups, and by 1998 joined the board of directors of Genetic Alliance, becoming President in 2002, and CEO in 2004. At Genetic Alliance, we expanded the methods, resources, and tools PXE International had developed so that all organizations could use them. We formally established the Genetic Alliance Registry and BioBank in 2003. We articulated the importance of collaboration among all stakeholders, including patients, clinicians, researchers, and policy makers. We established guidelines, principles, and trainings [6–9]. We enlisted ethicists, anthropologists, theologians, sociologists, and Barack Obama's campaign leaders to help us understand the importance of culture and the barriers between the stakeholders. We began to understand that cultural humility, whether about systemic racism, or the competitive culture of academic science, was critical to our having an impact in our quest to have people recognized as part of the team. Immense support from leaders at the Health Resources Services Administration (HRSA) allowed us to explore and add to the science of engagement [10–12].

Genetic Alliance has led the way in putting people—individuals, families, and communities—at the center of health research and services. We have contributed our leadership to help in the passage of the Genetic Information Nondiscrimination Act passed, the formation of the All of Us program, the establishment of the International Rare Disease Research Consortium, and many other international and national endeavors [13]. We influenced the inclusion of people-centered concepts and ideas such as those codified in the law through which the Food and Drug Administration gets it authority to oversee drug development: patient-focused drug development and real-world evidence [14]. We aren't satisfied with having a place at the table; we want to collaborate with others to decide where the table will be, who will be invited to it, what and how the meal will be served. People-centered, team science cannot be just given lip-service; there must be meaningful and dynamic actions.

Two recent projects of Genetic Alliance exemplify our deepening understand of what it means to be collaborative, to lead teams, and play well. The first is our involvement in PCORnet, the clinical research network of the Patient Centered

Outcomes Research Institute. For 5 years, Genetic Alliance served with Harvard Pilgrim Health Care Institute and Duke Clinical Research Institute as the PCORnet Coordinating Center. In that role, we led the engagement work. A wonderful outcome of that work is the Engagement Assessment Tool [15]. This tool is designed to guide stakeholders, investigators, and other contributors throughout a collaborative research process. These engagement steps, processes, and metrics can help develop partnerships and meet project objectives. It details elements for effective engagement, key steps, process and products, and monitoring and metrics for every stage of research: research planning, design, and proposal development, research implementation, and dissemination of results.

The other project is a long-time project of Genetic Alliance: our registry. As stated above, we established our cross-condition registry in 2003, before the advent of the necessary technology that puts people in control of their data. Though we expanded and customized various off-the-shelf software, we could never find a way to give people complete control of their data. Finally, in early 2019, we partnered with LunaDNA to give people the tools to "keep a string on their data," to know who is using it, and to share in the ecosystem of the benefits – from discovery to sharing in the actual profits. Individuals who share their PRO, their EHR (we have connections to 89% of the EHR portals natinally) and/or genomic information own LunaDNA [16, 17]. We have many communities using this system we call the Promise to Engage Everyone Responsibly (PEER), e.g., disease advocacy groups, environmental organizations, racial justice communities, professional societies, national umbrella organizations. With Luna, we have developed a system to validate PRO in a short time, giving communities the power to determine even the instruments that represent their needs. We now have the tools to put people in the center, on the team, making decisions about what they need most, setting priorities for research, collaborating on studies. A number of biopharmaceutical companies have begun to use our system so that communities can be formed even from rudimentary social networks, and clinical studies can be done remotely, where people live, work, and play. This is broadly engaged team science.

Transforming Systems Requires Transforming Ourselves

We who seek meaningful change must understand what it means to transform systems, dissolve boundaries, and promote the process of openness. We must also understand that to transform systems, we must start with our very person, our own organism. Such work calls us, both personally and professionally, to explore the deepest truths about ourselves and the systems we impact. After all, if I am not open and vulnerable, clear and explicit, then I cannot expect the systems in which I work to be collaborative and transformative. For myself, I make sure that I spend time and attention on becoming more aware: of myself, my choices, my actions, and my impact. I know that to do this well I must understand what I fear and to gently face those fears.

Changing the status quo, coming into contact with the boundaries of broken systems, with seemingly paternalistic or elitist leaders who may not want to change, requires that I become aware of my own resistance, fear, and prejudice. My awareness leads me to choices, instead of staying in the same groove and not seeing options. This allows me to trust my teammates, and to trust the process of working together. Without trust, we cannot build teams and transform systems. I work with many groups and families who experience a lot of suffering and death. I am often reminded of the poet Mary Oliver's question: *Tell me, what is it you plan to do with your one wild and precious life?* If each of us live into that question, we will show up more fully with one another, and especially for those we seek to help.

References

1. Mackta JS, Weiss JO (1996) Starting and sustaining genetic support groups. Johns Hopkins University Press, United States
2. Bercovitch L, Schepps B, Koelliker S, Magro C, Terry S, Lebwohl M (2003) Mammographic findings in pseudoxanthoma elasticum. J Am Acad Dermatol 48(3):359–366. https://doi.org/10.1067/mjd.2003.173. PMID: 12637915
3. Bercovitch RS, Januario JA, Terry SF, Boekelheide K, Podis AD, Dupuy DE, Bercovitch LG (2005) Testicular microlithiasis in association with pseudoxanthoma elasticum. Radiology 237(2):550–554. https://doi.org/10.1148/radiol.2372041136. PMID: 16244264
4. Bergen AA, Plomp AS, Schuurman EJ, Terry SF, Breuning M, Dauwerse H, Swart J, Kool M, van Soest S, Baas F, ten Brink JB, de Jong PT (2000) Mutations in ABCC6 cause pseudoxanthoma elasticum. Nat Genet 25(2):228–231. https://doi.org/10.1038/76109. PMID: 10835643
5. Le Saux O, Urban Z, Tschuch C, Csiszar K, Bacchelli B, Quaglino D, Pasquali-Ronchetti I, Pope FM, Richards A, Terry S, Bercovitch L, de Paepe A, Boyd CD (2000) Mutations in a gene encoding an ABC transporter cause pseudoxanthoma elasticum. Nat Genet 25(2):223–227. https://doi.org/10.1038/76102. PMID: 10835642
6. Terry SF, Horn EJ, Scott J, Terry PF (2011) Genetic Alliance Registry and BioBank: a novel disease advocacy-driven research solution. Per Med 8(2):207–213. https://doi.org/10.2217/pme.11.1. PMID: 29783403
7. Terry SF, Terry PF, Rauen KA, Uitto J, Bercovitch LG (2007) Advocacy groups as research organizations: the PXE International example. Nat Rev Genet 8(2):157–164. https://doi.org/10.1038/nrg1991. PMID: 17230202
8. Kaye J, Terry SF, Juengst E, Coy S, Harris JR, Chalmers D, Dove ES, Budin-Ljøsne I, Adebamowo C, Ogbe E, Bezuidenhout L, Morrison M, Minion JT, Murtagh MJ, Minari J, Teare H, Isasi R, Kato K, Rial-Sebbag E, Marshall P, Koenig B, Cambon-Thomsen A (2018) Including all voices in international data-sharing governance. Hum Genomics 7;12(1):13. https://doi.org/10.1186/s40246-018-0143-9. PMID: 29514717; PMCID: PMC5842530
9. Terry SF (2017) The study is open: Participants are now recruiting investigators. Sci Transl Med 4;9(371):eaaf1001. https://doi.org/10.1126/scitranslmed.aaf1001. PMID: 28053150
10. Rangi SK, Terry SF (2014) Genetic testing and native peoples: the call for community-based participatory research. Genet Test Mol Biomarkers 18(8):531–532. https://doi.org/10.1089/gtmb.2014.1557. PMID: 25089910
11. Mena C, Terry S (2018) No seat at the recommendations table? Genet Test Mol Biomarkers 22(1):3–4. https://doi.org/10.1089/gtmb.2017.29039.sjt. PMID: 29345983
12. Terry SF (2017) Research for the people by the people. Genet Test Mol Biomarkers 21(9):521–522. https://doi.org/10.1089/gtmb.2017.29034.sjt. PMID: 28915083

13. Terry SF (2009) Genetic information nondiscrimination act insurance protections issued. Genet Test Mol Biomarkers 13(6):709–710. https://doi.org/10.1089/gtmb.2009.1507. PMID: 20001579

14. Prescription Drug User Fee Act (PDUFA) (1992) United States of America

15. Engagement Tool and Resource Repository. PCORI. https://www.pcori.org/engagement/engagement-resources/Engagement-Tool-Resource-Repository/engagement-assessment-tool

16. Kain R, Kahn S, Thompson D, Lewis D, Barker D, Bustamante C, Cabou C, Casdin A, Garcia F, Paragas J, Patrinos A, Rajagopal A, Terry SF, Van Zeeland A, Yu E, Erlich Y, Barry D (2019) Database shares that transform research subjects into partners. Nat Biotechnol 37(10):1112–1115. https://doi.org/10.1038/s41587-019-0278-9. PMID: 31537916

17. Fox K (2020) The illusion of inclusion - The "All of Us" research program and indigenous peoples' DNA. N Engl J Med 383(5):411–413. https://doi.org/10.1056/NEJMp1915987. PMID: 32726527

Chapter 3
Broadly Engaged Team Science in Neonatal Research

Jonathan M. Davis

Abstract Unlike treatments used in older children and adults, most medications administered to preterm neonates lack robust data to support their safety and efficacy. Moreover, no new drugs have been developed to substantially improve survival and outcome for preterm neonates since pulmonary surfactant almost 30 years ago. The International Neonatal Consortium (INC) was established in 2015 to address key regulatory gaps and provide a more global and structured approach to neonatal drug development. Initially, the INC is focusing on two therapeutic areas (seizures, chronic lung injury) and two cross-cutting projects (clinical pharmacology, data standards) expected to benefit all therapeutic areas. This work will advance regulatory science by focusing on the needs of the neonate and will add value by increasing the predictability of the regulatory path for neonatal medicines, creating an evidence base to enhance prevention and treatment strategies, and demonstrating approaches that are transferable between therapeutic areas.

Keywords International Neonatal Consortium (INC) · Therapeutic orphans · Drug evaluation in neonates · Standardizing neonatal data · Neonatal research studies · Neonatal drug development

Approximately 200,000 neonates born annually in the United States require admission to a neonatal intensive care unit for treatment of prematurity, costing more than $25 billion per year [1]. Preterm neonates are at significant risk of serious morbidity and mortality that can affect them for life. Unlike treatments used in older children and adults, most medications administered to preterm neonates lack robust data to support their safety and efficacy, with 60–90% not approved by most global regulatory agencies for the prescribed indication. No new drugs have been developed to substantially improve survival and outcome for preterm neonates since the introduction of pulmonary surfactant almost 30 years ago [2]. The smallest and most critically ill neonates may be exposed to more than 60 separate drugs, with the most

J. M. Davis (✉)
Tufts Clinical and Translational Science Institute; Tufts Children's Hospital, Boston, MA, USA
e-mail: jdavis@tuftsmedicalcenter.org

© The Author(s), under exclusive license to Springer Nature Switzerland AG 2022
D. Lerner et al. (eds.), *Broadly Engaged Team Science in Clinical and Translational Research*, https://doi.org/10.1007/978-3-030-83028-1_3

19

preterm neonates receiving the greatest number of medications [3]. This is why neonates have been called "therapeutic orphans" by many clinicians who care for these patients. Serious adverse drug reactions from single or multiple drugs can significantly increase morbidity and mortality resulting in short- and long-term adverse consequences [4]. In addition, there are relatively few drug formulations that are safe for neonates, which means drugs suspended in potentially toxic alcohol and/or propylene glycol (as preservatives) are routinely administered to the smallest and most vulnerable patients [5].

Drug development for this population has been slow due to both economic and methodological challenges. These include a small market (which limits a drug's commercial potential) and barriers to research such as the low prevalence of certain diseases, the potential risks to patients (and potential manufacturer liability), the absence of appropriate animal models, hard to define safety and efficacy criteria, numerous complexities associated with study design and outcomes measurement, and the lengthy durations of follow-up needed to determine neurobehavioral outcomes. As a result, each preterm neonate is in effect being enrolled in an uncontrolled and unapproved clinical trial that will not yield data of substantial value.

Formation of the International Neonatal Consortium (INC)

In order to address this key regulatory gap and provide a more global and structured approach to neonatal drug development, the Food and Drug Administration (FDA) helped establish the International Neonatal Consortium (INC) in May 2015. INC is supervised by the non-profit Critical Path Institute (C-Path) and functions within a "precompetitive space" to promote unique collaborations between companies that would normally be competitors while addressing the need for measurement and assessment of clinical outcomes in neonates through teams that share data and expertise to advance regulatory science. The work of INC has grown to engage all the key stakeholders involved in the drug development paradigm (Fig. 3.1) [6].

INC started with a grant from the FDA as regulators recognized that neonates were being excluded from the drug development paradigm and the situation was unlikely to change without regulatory intervention. The FDA then reached out to Health Canada, the European Medicines Agency, and other global regulatory agencies to better standardize approaches to neonatal drug development and approval worldwide. These agencies engaged in discussions with other key stakeholders (selected by appointment, nomination, and invitation to join INC) who were motivated to have direct and productive discussions with regulators due to legislative requirements for sponsors to conduct neonatal drug development programs. INC was able to have these discussions by being product agnostic. This allowed regulators to interact with industry, academic researchers, clinical neonatologists, nurses, and families without the risk of perceived conflict of interest. Meaningful involvement of multiple key stakeholders is essential as safe, ethical, and effective clinical trials cannot be conducted without all their participation. Each stakeholder group,

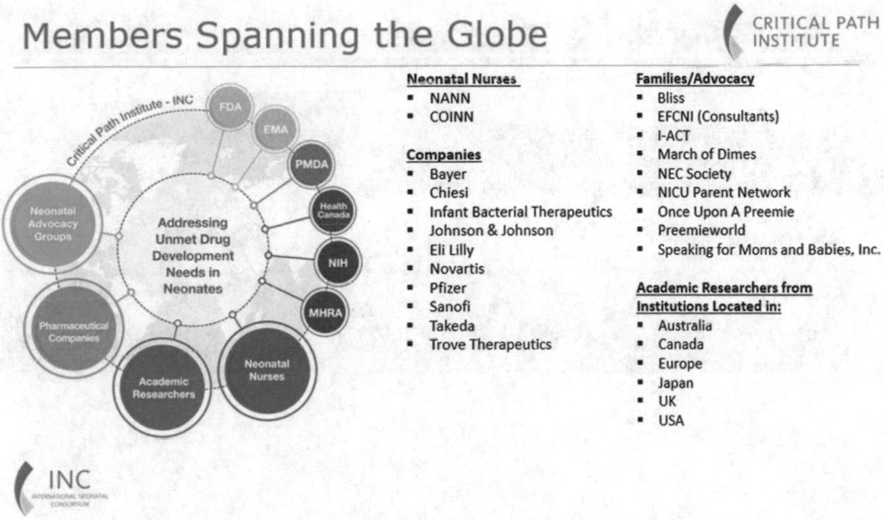

Fig. 3.1 Membership in INC: (300 members, 77 academic institutions, 25 countries); *FDA* Food and Drug Administration, *EMA* European Medicines Agency, *PMDA* Pharmaceuticals and Medical Devices Agency of Japan, *NIH* National Institutes of Health [6]

especially parents of premature infants, brings a unique perspective which must be better understood by other participants. Standardized approaches are needed as much as possible across many populations and cultures so clinical trials can be conducted in a similar fashion and high-quality data can be generated and compared. Key to the success of INC is dedicated project management to convene workshops, which drive the production of deliverables, including qualified biomarkers and clinical outcome assessments, regulatory-endorsed clinical trial simulation tools, data standards, and clinical trial databases published in a wide variety of medical journals.

Initial Cross-Cutting Themes of INC

During the early stages of INC, a Coordinating Committee was established as well as a governance structure (Fig. 3.2). INC stakeholders identified critical needs for the therapeutic areas in the neonatal intensive care unit that contributed most strongly to adverse neonatal outcomes. Priorities were established then voted on, with parents having the same vote as a neonatologist. Parents who have had an infant in the NICU are embedded throughout INC as they have particularly important information to provide to all participants. From these needs assessments, an initial set of INC priorities were selected. Two of the priorities focused on therapeutic areas (seizures, chronic lung injury) and two priorities were cross-cutting projects (clinical pharmacology, data standards) expected to benefit all therapeutic areas.

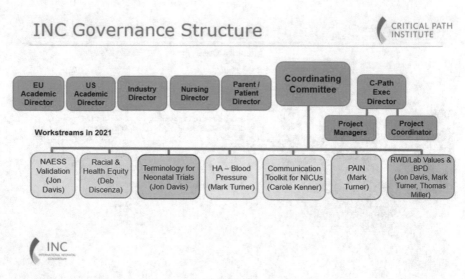

Fig. 3.2 INC Governance Structure: *EU* European Union, *US* United States, *BPD* bronchopulmonary dysplasia, *Clin Pharm* clinical pharmacology, *HA* hemodynamic adaptation, *ROP* retinopathy of prematurity, *NEC* necrotizing enterocolitis, *Comms* communications [6]

The first cross-cutting project, clinical pharmacology, involved improving our understanding of drug evaluation in neonates, taking into account organ immaturity and evolving regulatory guidance [6]. This included the urgent need to develop a more unified and consistent approach to studying new and existing drugs in neonates. It was also consistent with INC's key goals of sharing and enhancing best practices for designing and implementing clinical trials (e.g., how to choose the optimal outcome measures), using existing data (e.g., how and when to perform extrapolation procedures), and pharmacokinetic studies (e.g., when to use opportunistic assessment of scavenged blood samples and determining sample sizes for population pharmacokinetic studies). Based on its research, INC's clinical pharmacology group developed a comprehensive white paper to guide neonatal clinical trials of drugs and biologics – particularly early phase studies [7]. Key points include: the need to base drug development on neonatal physiology and pharmacology while making the most of knowledge acquired in other settings; the central role of families in research; and the value of the whole neonatal team in the design, implementation, and interpretation of studies. This white paper has already facilitated the successful completion of clinical trials of drugs in neonates by informing regulators, sponsors, and the neonatal community of existing good practice. In addition, this document is being used by global regulators to improve guidance for sponsors and investigators who are developing new drugs for testing in neonates and by regulators and legislators in many countries to pass legislation to promote neonatal and pediatric drug development efforts.

The second cross-cutting project established data standards for clinical trials in neonates. The relatively small number of neonates with rare diseases and the large number of covariates require data to be pooled across many populations and countries. Pooling data on a global scale requires the use of shared or standardized definitions of data and databases that can be queried consistently (i.e., interoperable databases). Federating databases that contain routinely collected harmonized and standardized data will provide useful information on the natural history of disease, biomarkers, clinical end points, standards of care, normal laboratory values, and long-term follow-up of clinically meaningful outcomes. An enormous amount of neonatal data is continually generated and stored in databases around the world. These data serve a variety of purposes, including clinical care, benchmarking, quality improvement, advocacy, health services evaluation, and research. With a focus on clinical research, INC is tapping existing resources to explore how they can be interrogated to improve the design and execution of trials, including the consistent, timely, and reproducible identification and reporting of efficacy and safety outcomes. An overview of selected databases reveals considerable variation in definitions, terminologies, methodologies, and organization of data elements. As a first step towards standardizing neonatal data, a core set of data elements and their associated descriptors were identified that could be productively and routinely collected in neonatal data collection platforms or neonatal research studies across the globe [8]. A framework for future standardization of neonatal data will be developed by collaborative INC working groups to facilitate alignment of current data efforts while leveraging these platforms to enhance global collaborations in future drug development trials.

Key Deliverables of INC

Stakeholders working within INC have published a number of important manuscripts and formally responded to government requests for information. These actions have had significant impact on neonatal drug development processes, including: (1) establishing a global neonatal research community [6], (2) supplying objective expert information to governments, (3) aligning on pharmacologic considerations for neonatal trials [7], (4) promoting data sharing to support new drug development tools [7], (5) innovating the design of neonatal clinical trials [9], (6) determining the normal range of blood pressures in neonates and the optimal methods of measurement [10], (7) assessing safety signals in neonatal clinical trials [11], (8) standardizing safety reporting in neonatal clinical trials where background rates of complications are already high [12], (9) developing terminology and data standards with the National Cancer Institute, (10) assessing long-term neurodevelopmental outcome in neonatal drug trials [13], and many others dealing with complications in the lung, intestines, brain, and eyes in preterm neonates [8, 14–16].

INC Is Advancing Neonatal Regulatory Science

Advancing neonatal regulatory science is essential for the timely development of new treatments and for improved use of existing drugs for neonates. The enormous challenges to conducting clinical studies in neonates, particularly preterm neonates who often have a variety of rare diseases, can only be addressed through concerted and coordinated efforts of all stakeholders. INC has advanced regulatory science by focusing on the needs of the neonate and will add value by increasing the predictability of the regulatory path for neonatal medicines, creating an evidence base to enhance prevention and treatment strategies, and demonstrating approaches that are transferable between therapeutic areas. This is a unique example of a regulatory agency taking a different approach to engaging stakeholders and how family members and other experts must learn to interact in new ways. INC is also an example of how the drug development process can be transformed to include greater stakeholder involvement.

References

1. Davis JM, Connor EM, Wood AJ (2012) The need for rigorous evidence on medication use in preterm infants: is it time for a neonatal rule? JAMA 308:1435–1436
2. Laughon MM, Avant D, Tripathi N et al (2014) Drug labeling and exposure in neonates. JAMA Pediatr 168:130–136
3. Kumar P, Walker JK, Hurt KM, Bennett KM, Grosshans N, Fotis MA (2008) Medication use in the neonatal intensive care unit: current patterns and off-label use of parenteral medications. J Pediatr 152:412–415
4. Moore TJ, Weiss SR, Kaplan S, Blaisdell CJ (2002) Reported adverse drug events in infants and children under 2 years of age. Pediatrics 110:e53
5. Buckley LA, Salunke S, Thompson K, Baer G, Fegley D, Turner MA (2018) Challenges and strategies to facilitate formulation development of pediatric drug products: Safety qualification of excipients. Int J Pharm 536:563–569
6. Davis JM, Turner MA (2015) Global collaboration to develop new and existing drugs for neonates. JAMA Pediatr 169:887–888
7. Ward RM, Benjamin D, Barrett JS, Allegaert K, Portman R, Davis JM, Turner MA (2017) Safety, dosing, and pharmaceutical quality for studies that evaluate medicinal products (including biological products) in neonates. Pediatr Res 81:692–711
8. Costeloe K, Turner MA, Padula MA, et al (2018) Sharing data to accelerate medicine development and improve neonatal care: Data standards and harmonized definitions. J Pediatr 203:437–441.e1
9. Soul JS, Pressler R, Allen M et al (2019) Recommendations for the design of therapeutic trials for neonatal seizures. Pediatr Res 85:943–954
10. Dionne JM, Bremner SA, Baygani SK et al (2020) Proper method of blood pressure measurement in neonates and infants: a systematic review and analysis. J Pediatr. (in press)
11. Salaets T, Turner MA, Short M et al (2019) Development of a neonatal adverse event severity scale through a Delphi consensus approach. Arch Dis Child 104:1167–1173
12. Davis JM, Baer GR, McCune S, et al (2020) Standardizing safety assessment and reporting for neonatal clinical trials. J Pediatr 219:243–249.e1

13. Marlow N, Doyle LW, Anderson P et al (2019) Assessment of long-term neurodevelopmental outcome following trials of medicinal products in newborn infants. Pediatr Res 86:567–572
14. Steinhorn R, Davis JM, Göpel W, et al (2017) Chronic pulmonary insufficiency of prematurity: developing optimal endpoints for drug development. J Pediatr 191:15–21.e1
15. Caplan MS, Underwood MA, Modi N, et al (2019) Necrotizing Enterocolitis: using regulatory science and drug development to improve outcomes. J Pediatr 212:208–215.e1
16. Smith LEH, Hellström A, Stahl A et al (2019) Development of a retinopathy of prematurity activity scale and clinical outcome measures for use in clinical trials. JAMA Ophthalmol 137:305–311

Chapter 4
The Changing Role of Patient Advocates in Cancer Clinical Trials

Susan K. Parsons

Abstract The stunning improvements in cancer outcomes over the past 60 years have been built on a strong foundation of formal cancer clinical trials. These trials serve as the conduit to new therapies, and their success depends on robust collaboration between researchers, health professionals, patients, and most recently recognized, patient advocates. Traditionally, patient advocates in cancer clinical trials have been individuals with an intimate knowledge of what it means to have a cancer diagnosis, either directly as a survivor of cancer, or collaterally, as a family member or close friend of someone with cancer. This chapter highlights the Southwestern Oncology Group (SWOG), which was the first to incorporate patient advocates into the clinical trials structure in the early 1990s. Since then, patient advocacy at SWOG has evolved considerably and now includes formal training to help advocates work effectively in multi-disciplinary research teams.

Keywords Cancer patient advocacy · Cancer patient advocate · Southwestern Oncology Group · SWOG · Cancer clinical trials structure

The stunning improvements in cancer outcomes over the past 60 years have been built on a strong foundation of formal cancer clinical trials. This is especially true in pediatric oncology, where clinical trial participation among newly diagnosed patients is approximately 80%. As Danielle Leach, career-long patient advocate, current Chief of Community and Government Relations for the National Brain Tumor Society, former director of Government Relations for the St. Baldrick's Foundation, and devoted mother of her late son, Mason, reminds us, "In the 1950's, almost all of the kids diagnosed with cancer died. Because of research, today about 90% of kids with the most common type of cancer [acute lymphoblastic leukemia] will live." She goes on to say that "for many other types, progress is limited and for some kids there is no hope for a cure. Our job is not done…[1]."

S. K. Parsons (✉)
Institute for Clinical Research and Health Policy Studies, Tufts Medical Center, Boston, MA, USA
e-mail: sparsons@tuftsmedicalcenter.org

© The Author(s), under exclusive license to Springer Nature Switzerland AG 2022
D. Lerner et al. (eds.), *Broadly Engaged Team Science in Clinical and Translational Research*, https://doi.org/10.1007/978-3-030-83028-1_4

27

Clinical trials serve as the principal pathway to experimental therapies, often providing hope for disease control not realized with conventional therapy. Through rigorous development, novel therapies must demonstrate both safety and tolerability as well as efficacy versus standard care/treatments. The successful implementation of clinical trials depends on robust collaboration between researchers, health professionals, patients, and patient advocates.

A Brief History of Cancer Clinical Trials

For nearly 70 years, the National Cancer Institute (NCI) has provided the infrastructure and support for cancer clinical trials in the United States. Federal underwriting of the cost of new therapies has been essential—because the drug development process is lengthy (estimated 12–18 years), expensive, and often fraught with failure. In a 2019 report, the success rate of clinical trials was only 5–14% in the period from 2006–2014 [2].

Early on in the development of cancer clinical trials, several NCI-sponsored cooperative groups were formed, primarily based on geography and/or patient age (i.e., adult or pediatric). These cooperative groups, now referred to as "legacy" groups, initially fostered multi-institutional clinical trial collaborations and later also encouraged multi-disciplinary involvement including the medical, nursing, psychology/behavioral science, cancer control, and cancer care delivery fields.

In 1971, then President Nixon signed into law the National Cancer Act as a declaration of war against cancer. The goal of the legislation was to accelerate research on the development of new therapies in order to reduce the suffering and premature mortality from cancer. While federal funds for cancer research expanded considerably over the next 40 years, progress in both elucidating the cause(s) and eradicating the disease was generally deemed to be too slow.

In 2010 the Institute of Medicine (IOM) issued a report entitled, "A National Cancer Clinical Trials System for the 21st Century [3]." The report outlined steps to improve the speed and efficiency of trials from design, to launch, to conduct. These steps included: optimal use of scientific innovation; improved selection, prioritization, support, and completion of clinical trials; and finally, fostering expanded involvement of both patients and physicians throughout the clinical trials development process. By 2014, the National Clinical Trials Network was established (Fig. 4.1). Several of the original cooperative groups were merged and renamed to remove reference solely to geography [4].

Included in the 2014 re-engineering of the cancer clinical trials structure was the creation of the Clinical Trials and Translational Research Advisory Council, reporting to the NCI director. Council members included clinical trialists, industry representatives, and patient advocates, to enhance the design and conduct of clinical trials.

NCI National Clinical Trials Network Structure

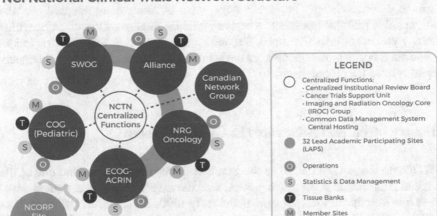

Fig. 4.1 The National Cancer Institute (NCI) National Clinical Trials Network Structure

Cancer Patient Advocacy Has Taken Many Forms

Traditionally, cancer patient advocates have been individuals with an intimate knowledge of what it means to have a cancer diagnosis, either directly as a survivor of cancer, or collaterally, as a family member or close friend of someone with cancer. Some of the most poignant and powerful patient advocacy has been delivered by bereft family members who want future cancer patients to have better experiences than their loved ones did—through more effective treatments, improvements in care delivery, enhanced support (e.g., palliative or hospice care), or advances in scientific discovery. Advocates routinely serve as fundraisers, lobbyists, grassroots organizers, and spokespeople for the cancer community. Examples of advocacy organizations include those that are: (1) disease-specific, such as the Susan B. Komen Foundation (breast cancer) or the Leukemia & Lymphoma Society (blood cancers); (2) age-based, such as Alex's Lemonade Stand (pediatric oncology); or (3) cancer-wide, such as the American Cancer Society. Advocates like Danielle Leach have been able to marshal their personal devastation into action while also encouraging others to participate in advocacy roles, bringing ever-fresh voice to the process.

At times, cancer patient advocates have served as teachers. They have paid close attention to the collective use of language in study materials, such as consent documents, information sheets, and publications to ensure they are clear, inclusive, and sensitive to the patient experience. Advocates have discouraged the use of possessive pronouns to describe cancer, symptoms, or outcomes (e.g., "his" cancer), pointing out that patients do not become the cancer and do not want to "own" or be responsible for its sequelae. Similarly, advocates have urged researchers not to use verbs to describe changes in disease stage, such as "the patient relapsed" or "the patient failed frontline treatment." They suggest "the disease recurred" or "frontline therapy was not effective," instead. Beyond simply semantics, this attention to language helps health professionals keep the patient at the center of their work, uniquely separate from the disease itself.

History of Patient Advocates in Clinical Trials

SWOG, previously referred to as the Southwest Oncology Group, and one of the original NCI-funded cooperative groups, was the first to incorporate patient advocates into the clinical trials structure in the early 1990s. By 2008, each disease committee within SWOG had one to two assigned advocates to work with study committees on the development and conduct of clinical trials. The vice chair of the advocates' committee, who herself is a career-long advocate, has been a member of the SWOG lymphoma committee for 10 years. She argues that having patient advocates involved in clinical trials development and execution is not new. What is new is the concerted effort to help clinicians and non-clinician members *effectively engage* patients and other stakeholders.

In 2016 the SWOG team was awarded a Eugene Washington Patient-Centered Outcomes Research Institute (PCORI) Engagement Award, which led to the creation of formal training for patient advocates. The goal of the training was to help advocates work effectively in multi-disciplinary research teams, learning when and how to speak up. The field guide, entitled "TeamScience@SWOG," and disseminated on the SWOG member website, contains five modules for members of the clinical trials team, including three specifically tailored for patient advocates to take them from idea generation through implementation and results-sharing [5]. Modules were also developed to help clinician leaders understand how best to work with advocates. Historically, clinical trials leadership was reserved for more senior members of the disease or discipline groups. Within SWOG, senior members had "grown up" within a culture of partnership with patient advocates. Increasingly, junior members are being developed to lead clinical trials. The specific training offered through the Team Science field guide, while useful for all investigators, is especially important for these new/junior investigators who may not have prior experience working with advocates.

In addition to availability of training modules, a new framework has been developed to formally integrate advocates in the clinical trials development process (Fig. 4.2). The previous structure, shown in black lettering, was largely driven by clinician researchers, whereas the revised process, shown in blue lettering, reflects increased collaboration and more active participation of advocates. The new framework ensures the role of the advocate is incorporated into every step of the trial process from development to dissemination.

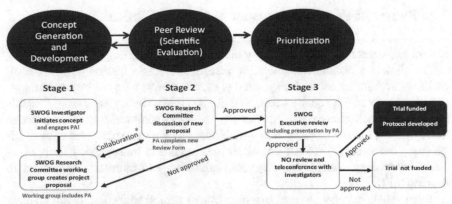

*Training and communication for Patient Advocate (PA), Principal Investigators, Protocol Coordinators, and Executive Leadership
SWOG, Southwestern Oncology Group; NCI, National Cancer Institute

Fig. 4.2 SWOG Researcher-Advocate Engagement Framework, adapted from Deverka PA et al. [6], highlights patient advocates' (PA) evolving role

Incorporating Patient Advocates into Designing and Implementing Clinical Trials

In the planning of a recent trial involving novel, costly new therapies, a SWOG lymphoma committee advocate recommended the following considerations about broaching broad financial themes with patients. This advocate reminds us that patients or their caregivers might need assistance to anticipate and manage short- or long-term financial, school or workplace distress during enrollment. In materials prepared for the currently accruing clinical trial, she urges us not to assume there is not moderate to severe cancer-related distress, but also not to assume that patients in moderate to severe distress cannot participate in trials. "Do all you can to make it possible for them to participate. Be prepared with referral resources for patients and caregivers." To address her latter point, she also assembled resources about health care costs for patients and their providers to use to enhance understanding about the potential financial impact of trial participation. These resources have been posted on the study website, utilized in staff training, and shared with trial participants.

Beyond the respect such behaviors demonstrate, they also directly benefit the conduct and success of the trial. In this particular case, clinical trial investigators were concerned about potential "randomization regret," i.e., if the patient were randomly assigned to the study arm in which the commercially available drug was used. Drugs that are commercially available are not provided to study participants free of charge through the trial, but rather, subject to available coverage through the patient's insurance. Thus, assignment to the commercially available drug might result in higher patient cost than assignment to the experimental arm in which study drug was provided at no cost to the study participant. Randomization regret can lead to differential treatment group drop out and imbalance between study arms, which can result in biased findings. By calling attention to the topic of cost and by assembling resources for participants across study arms, these issues have been reduced.

The Future of Patient Advocacy in Cancer Clinical Trials

Patient advocates have an increasingly integral role in designing and implementing cancer clinical trials and disseminating results. Advocates remind us that not all patients have similar access to, knowledge of, or comfort with the health care system. They may not be equally trusting of clinical trials, shying away from "experimentation" or being treated as a "guinea pig." Minority communities still reverberate from previous failures of protection—including government-sponsored clinical trials (e.g., Tuskegee) [7]. To address disparities in clinical trials participation, especially in minority communities, targeted education and outreach are needed to develop trust.

Even among patients inclined to participate in clinical trials, it may not be clear who to ask or how to ask for help. Patients may not understand how trials are designed or run, what treatments they will get or what follow-up is required. Advocates' experience and expertise means that they can guide patients through clinical trial information with care and concern. Patient education materials are often inadequate, and onsite staff can help usher patients through treatment. Some centers rely on lay navigators, serving as advocates, to work with the clinical team and the clinical trials staff to ensure adequate understanding and adherence.

Patient advocates serve as teachers, students, and partners. As the SWOG group chair, Charles Blanke reminds us, "Advocates make our trials better. They help ensure our work is relevant and realistic and efficient. We want our trials to open and close quickly and, in the end, have a big positive impact on people with cancer. Advocates get us there [8]."

References

1. Leach D (2014) What I told our senators about childhood cancer. St. Baldrick's Foundation: Conquer Childhood Cancers
2. Wong CH, Siah KW, Lo AW (2019) Estimation of clinical trial success rates and related parameters. Biostatistics 20(2):273–286. https://doi.org/10.1093/biostatistics/kxx069
3. Institute of Medicine Committee on Cancer Clinical T, the NCICGP (2010) In: Nass SJ, Moses HL, Mendelsohn J (eds) A national cancer clinical trials system for the 21st century: reinvigorating the NCI cooperative group program. National Academies Press (US) Copyright 2010 by the National Academy of Sciences. All rights reserved., Washington (DC). https://doi.org/10.17226/12879
4. NCI National Clinical Trials Network Structure. https://www.cancer.gov/sites/g/files/xnrzdm211/files/styles/cgov_enlarged/public/cgov_infographic/2019-07/NCTN_Clinical_Trials_Network.gif?itok=fL234Ga4. Accessed 15 Jan 2021
5. SWOG (2018) TeamScience@SWOG: Field Guide. pcori.org
6. Deverka PA, Bangs R, Kreizenbeck K, Delaney DM, Hershman DL, Blanke CD, Ramsey SD (2018) A new framework for patient engagement in cancer clinical trials cooperative group studies. J Natl Cancer Inst 110(6):553–559. https://doi.org/10.1093/jnci/djy064
7. The Tuskegree Timeline (2020). https://www.cdc.gov/tuskegee/timeline.htm. Accessed 15 Jan 2021
8. SWOG Patient Advocate Resource Guide (2018). swog.org. Accessed 15 Jan 2021

Chapter 5
National Kidney Foundation (NKF) Patient Network

Silvia Ferrè, Silvia Titan, and Lesley A. Inker

Abstract The National Kidney Foundation (NKF) in partnership with Tufts Medical Center launched the first nationwide Chronic Kidney Disease (CKD) patient registry, known as the NKF Patient Network, powered by the combination of patient-entered data and clinical and laboratory data from electronic health records (EHR). In this chapter, we describe our sustainability plan to support the efficient operations and growth of this multifaceted and multi-stakeholder project. We present our strategy to select, engage, and evaluate different stakeholders and outline the governance structure that incorporates them in the oversight and development needed for the NKF Patient Network to grow and achieve its objectives.

Keywords Registry · Chronic kidney disease. · Patient-reported outcomes. · Electronic health records. · NKF Patient Network. · CKD registry. · RWD national registry. · Patient registry.

The Challenges in Chronic Kidney Disease (CKD) Clinical Management

Chronic kidney disease (CKD) is a growing worldwide public health problem, characterized by increasing prevalence, high cost, and poor outcomes [1]. In the United States (US), it affects 37 million adults [2, 3]. The poor outcomes include progression of kidney disease leading to chronic kidney failure, increased risk for acute

S. Ferrè
National Kidney Foundation, New York, NY, USA

S. Titan · L. A. Inker (✉)
Tufts Medical Center, Boston, MA, USA
e-mail: linker@tuftsmedicalcenter.org

© The Author(s), under exclusive license to Springer Nature Switzerland AG 2022
D. Lerner et al. (eds.), *Broadly Engaged Team Science in Clinical and Translational Research*, https://doi.org/10.1007/978-3-030-83028-1_5

kidney injury (AKI), cardiovascular disease (CVD), mortality, and a wide variety of other complications [1, 4]. CKD and Kidney Failure Replacement Therapy (KFRT) together impose a high financial burden, accounting for over \$110 billion in Medicare costs [5].

Despite the high prevalence and burden of the disease, approximately 90% of patients with CKD in the US are unaware of their condition because of the asymptomatic nature of the disease and under-diagnosis by health care professionals (HCPs) [6, 7]. Importantly, there are few specific and effective strategies to retard CKD progression and prevent or ameliorate complications [8]. With many other conditions, real-world evidence (RWE) studies based on real-world data (RWD), rather than data from regulated clinical trials, are becoming central to overcoming obstacles in care and disease management [9–13]. RWD are extracted from a broad range of sources, such as patient registries, health care databases, claims databases, and patient-generated data from wearables. Patient registries in particular form the foundation of population-based improvement activities that can lead to better care, because they facilitate identification of patients, capture clinical quality metrics, and track clinical outcomes [14, 15]. For kidney disease, RWD from electronic health records (EHR) have developed into population health strategies to improve CKD diagnosis and treatment. These include the CKD-Cure initiative, sponsored by Providence St. Joseph Health and the University of California, Los Angeles [16, 17], and the multicenter EHR-based CKD registry in Massachusetts [18]. However, no CKD registry so far includes both patient-reported and EHR data sources.

The National Kidney Foundation (NKF) in partnership with Tufts Medical Center launched the first nationwide CKD patient registry, known as the NKF Patient Network ("the Network"), powered by the unique combination of patient-entered data and clinical and laboratory data from EHR (Fig. 5.1). In this chapter, we describe our sustainability plan to support the efficient operations and growth of a multifaceted and multi-stakeholder project such as the NKF Patient Network. We present our strategy to select, engage, and evaluate the different stakeholders involved in this project, particularly people with kidney disease, HCPs, sponsor pharmaceutical companies, and the technology vendor. Lastly, we outline the governance structure that incorporates stakeholders in the oversight and development of future directions needed to help the Network grow and achieve its objectives.

The NKF Patient Network—Vision, Goals, and Architecture

Vision The NKF Patient Network is the first RWD national registry of adult patients with all stages of CKD that links patient-entered data on medical history, demographics, lifestyle, and perceptions with rigorous clinical and laboratory data from EHR. This novel structure has never been attempted before in CKD registries, because of the logistical challenges it poses. However, it offers multiple, unique opportunities, such as learning more about the natural history of the disease and advancing patient awareness, research, clinical care, and health policy making.

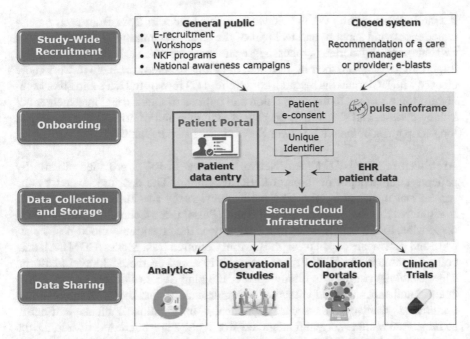

Fig. 5.1 Schema of the National Kidney Foundation (NKF) Patient Network. The NKF Patient Network is a national registry of adult patients with all stages of chronic kidney disease (CKD). Subjects are enrolled by wide recruitment methods, such as general market and integrated health networks. The registry links patient-entered data on their medical history, outcomes and preferences with clinical and laboratory data obtained from electronic health records (EHRs). Data is stored on a secured cloud platform maintained by Pulse Infoframe. Data is available to NKF Patient Network partners via customized portals and to the rest of community for multiple studies and clinical trials

Initially conceptualized by executives and experts at NKF and Tufts Medical Center, the Network is rapidly developing thanks to the support of multiple stakeholders. The NKF Patient Network will be rolled out in three phases. Phase 1 was completed in December 2020 and included: (1) the development of the technology infrastructure, and (2) a feasibility study phase that tested the linkage to EHR data with our first integrated health system partner Geisinger Health System. Phase 2 commenced in February 2021 and included the official national launch and a full-scale US national expansion, utilizing a broad marketing strategy integration We expect to recruit 1000 to 2000 US patients during the first year, and 10,000 to 50,000 US patients overall. Phase 3 will begin in the spring of 2022 with initiation of the international expansion and will include the Blue Button Medicare claims data integration in the US.

Goals The primary goal of the NKF Patient Network is to connect and educate patients with kidney disease while creating a database of patient-entered data and EHR data that helps patients, health care organizations, and multiple other stakeholders advance CKD diagnosis and treatment. Connecting patients and their families and other supports via the Network enables them to learn from each other's experiences, find support, and feel part of the CKD community. The availability of two data sources generates a robust aggregate database that: (1) helps patients derive important insights into their disease and, in doing so, empowers them to work more closely with HCPs and the research community; (2) reveals to HCPs and other organizations the barriers to the recognition and optimal evaluation and management of kidney disease, and sheds light on patient activities and priorities. The short- and long-term goals of the NKF Patient Network are listed in Table 5.1.

Architecture The NKF Patient Network consists of RWD provided directly by patients through input or through EHR integration. The data are owned by the patient and managed by the NKF with oversight by the Tufts Health Sciences Institutional Review Board. Pulse Infoframe (Pulse) is the technology vendor that is responsible for the development of the registry on their healthie™ cloud-based platform and data management using the OMOP Common Data Model (CDM). All data collected through the NKF Patient Network is stored on the healthie™ platform. The healthie™ platform is highly secure, utilizing Secure Sockets Layer (SSL)-enabled authentication and encrypted communications, and meets all international established standards for security of health information. Patients self-enroll at https://www.kidney.org/nkfpatientnetwork if they are interested in joining the program based on the information received through our recruitment channels, that include public relations, social media campaigns, and direct referral by HCPs at integrated health networks or medical centers (Fig. 5.1). Geisinger is one of the nation's most innovative health services organizations that serves more than 1.5 million patients in Pennsylvania and New Jersey. After signing an e-consent, patients are asked to fill in a questionnaire about their identification, demographics, diagnostics, and overall lifestyle. EHR integration occurs only if patients are affiliated with health care systems that are partners of the Network (i.e., Geisinger) or if they are Medicare beneficiaries who signed up for the Blue Button [19]. The list of variables collected in the registry have been decided and approved by two of the NKF Patient

Table 5.1 Goals of the National Kidney Foundation (NKF) Patient Network

Short-term goals
Foster patient disease awareness by educating both patients and their families through resources that are individualized to patients' stage of disease and related health conditions
Promote patients' interactions with each other as well as with their clinicians and the research community
Long-term goals
Create a robust database of patient outcomes, perceptions, priorities, and activities that will facilitate research, clinical care, and policy decisions to improve patients' experience and outcomes
Promote partnerships with health care organizations and health care systems to understand health care utilization data including cost of care for patients with CKD
Provide a large, diverse pool of patients for clinical trial recruitment, and input on patient-centered trial designs and opportunities for post-trial surveillance

Network's committees: the Data Input and Integration Committee and the Steering Committee. Data is available for analysis (e.g., descriptive statistics) to the partners of the NKF Patient Network via portals, dashboards, SAS server access, and/or reports, depending on contractual agreements. Research proposals by partners and outside organizations that require advanced statistical analysis will be submitted and approved according to the Data Use and Publications policy. The NKF Patient Network Governance oversees all operations related to the registry.

NKF Patient Network—Stakeholders

There are four stakeholders in the NKF Patient Network that present the greatest opportunities and challenges: people with kidney disease, the health systems (i.e., Geisinger, with others to follow) and HCPs, the sponsor pharmaceutical companies (i.e., Bayer, AstraZeneca, Boehringer Ingelheim, and Novartis), and the technology vendor (i.e., Pulse). Each stakeholder has different levels of interest in the project and ability to influence it which require *ad hoc* management models by NKF (Fig. 5.2). To present our management strategies, we addressed four main questions for each stakeholder: (1) Why is the stakeholder motivated to be engaged in the Network? (2) How have we designed the Network or its governance to engage the stakeholder in the Network and its operations? (3) How are we evaluating the stakeholder experience and participation? (4) How can the stakeholder impact research? Below we address each of these questions for these four key stakeholders.

People with Kidney Disease Getting diagnosed with a chronic disease that has poor outcomes and few effective therapeutic strategies can be isolating. A community such as the NKF Patient Network can be empowering and beneficial.

To further explore patients' motivations in engaging with the Network, the NKF team for Patient Engagement in collaboration with health economists at Pulse developed four patient journeys, one for each persona that we predicted will interact with the Network. The four personas were a patient recently diagnosed with early CKD, a patient with progressive CKD and comorbidities, a patient with ESRD receiving dialysis, and a patient with CKD who received a kidney transplant [20]. The journeys informed us that people with kidney disease will be motivated to engage with the Network because they will: i) have access to a one-stop shop for kidney resources that provide education, support, and tips on how to live a life with CKD, on dialysis, or after a kidney transplant, and how to maintain a healthy lifestyle; ii) gain the knowledge necessary to interface with primary care physicians and talk about kidney health wherever they are in the continuum of CKD; iii) stay up-to-date on both new and existing research and learn how to be a part of clinical trials and make a positive impact on treatment development; iv) connect to other people with kidney disease online and be notified about relevant events. To this end, the NKF Patient Network offers patients a user-friendly dashboard and secured portal with tooltips to assist navigation, a guide on how to enter their health data, and

Stakeholder Map

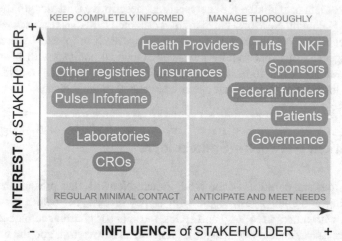

Fig. 5.2 Stakeholder Map. In green are stakeholders currently engaged in the NKF Patient Network; in orange are future stakeholders. The position of the labels within each quadrant reflects the level of influence and interest of the stakeholders. The text in grey indicates the level of management that the partnerships with stakeholders in each quadrant require

exclusive access to individualized education resources tailored to their disease stage via the NKF tool, Kidney Pathways [21]. Participants can connect to other people with similar kidney disease stage and demographic characteristics via online communities, forums, and blogs hosted on the platform and are notified of local events, latest findings in research, and clinical trial recruitment via newsletters. Moreover, patients receive patient-reported outcome measures (PROMs) and patient-reported experience measures (PREMs) on a regular frequency to explore and help prioritize symptomatology, preferences for and use of health care resources, lifestyle/diet modifications, changes in treatment, quality-of-life, and other measures.

Patient engagement and interaction with the platform are evaluated through satisfaction surveys, the number of patients who e-consented and who submitted PROMs and PREMs, the number of phone calls to the NKF Help Line to receive information and assistance with the Network, logins to the patient port, downloads and click-throughs of the education materials, and time spent on the pages.

We anticipate that the sense of community created among people with kidney disease, their families and HCPs will motivate the Network participants to share the initiative with friends, family members, and people that they may know who are impacted by kidney disease. This satisfaction will encourage participants to come back to the Network and share their data over time. Their outreach to fellow patients will ultimately lead to increased recruitment numbers. The Patient Advisory Group gathers constituents' input from comments that they receive from Network participants during NKF patient summits and other NKF events and brings this input to the attention of the Steering Committee.

The Health Systems and Health Care Professionals (HCPs) Health systems and HCPs are motivated to connect their patients to the Network because it provides insights on patient engagement with and perceptions of their disease and their care that are not routinely available through other means. In addition, it may allow for the evaluation of the implementation of evidence-based recommendations. Finally, the Network can improve the education of its patients by providing resources appropriate to their disease stage.

Not all health systems and HCPs receive the same amount of engagement with the Network. Health systems and HCPs that connect their patients with the Network are primarily passively engaged and derive benefit from their patients receiving individualized education. Health systems that contribute to both patient recruitment and EHR data integration additionally receive a clinician portal for data analysis, a dashboard for quick viewing of their patient data in eight charts, and patient-reported surveys (both PROMs and PREMs) for each of their patients, which can help them build or expand their kidney disease care management programs and report on quality measures. They also receive membership for one qualified executive on the Data Input and Integration Committee where they can impact research by proposing solutions and innovations to data collection and access.

Health systems that contribute to EHR data integration will be administered satisfaction surveys via the clinician portal every six months for the period of research contract asking about the usability of the platform and feasibility of recruitment. Individual HCPs can submit feedback to the NKF Patient Network research team via an online form available on the Network webpage or by calling the NKF Cares Help Line. The number of patients recruited per health system vs. from individual HCPs in the registry will ultimately inform NKF about the engagement of HCPs.

The Pharmaceutical Companies (Sponsors) Pharma sponsors are interested in the NKF Patient Network because it: i) provides insights on patient outcomes, perceptions, priorities and activities; ii) creates a diverse pool of patients with kidney disease for clinical trial recruitment and post-trial surveillance; iii) allows them to work with patient stakeholders on common projects.

Depending on the amount donated, sponsors receive a researcher portal with R or SAS interface for de-identified data analysis, a dashboard for quick data viewing in eight charts, aggregate patient-reported surveys, and/or subscription reports. Their satisfaction and participation is monitored quarterly upon submission of milestone reports, during monthly calls for the duration of the support period, and twice-a-year in-person meetings. Sponsors also receive recognition on all marketing materials and may also recommend one qualified executive on the Data Input and Integration Committee and Steering Committee. Through this committee, they can influence data collection by suggesting new variables to be collected, e.g., exposure to new medications, and can promote patient recruitment via their sale force. Pharma sponsors have been excluded intentionally from the Data Use and Publications Committee to prevent them from steering research towards topics of their interest.

The Technology Vendor (Pulse Infoframe) Pulse has created more than 40 registries that power research in the fields of cancer and rare diseases worldwide. Their healthie™ platform was designed to enable connectivity across stakeholder communities, creating the opportunity to share knowledge and inform new therapy. Pulse's motivations to participate in the NKF Patient Network are to: i) gain expertise in building registries for common, chronic diseases, such as CKD, and improve the platform with new functionalities for patients' and other stakeholders' engagement; ii) acquire visibility nationwide for RWE studies; iii) become the data hub for the Network.

Pulse is central to the development and ongoing organization of the Network. The Pulse team works in collaboration with the Technology Committee to work on solutions for data integration, content management models, and patient engagement. Furthermore, it is receiving recognition in all marketing materials directed to people with kidney disease and health care providers.

The experience of Pulse with the project and its participation are monitored from a strategic perspective via weekly calls with Pulse senior leadership and from an operational perspective via weekly calls with its director of operations.

As leader in the field of RWD, Pulse can impact the research done using the Network data through its representative on the Data Input and Integration Committee. The Pulse constituent can propose new data sources to integrate with the Network and new strategies to aid data viewing and reporting for all Network partners.

NKF Patient Network—Future Stakeholders

Once the Network is successfully implemented and ample data is available on the platform, we will be positioned to engage with the following stakeholders relevant to our long-term goals (Table 5.1 and Fig. 5.2):

Laboratories Testing laboratories, such as LabCorp, have access to laboratory data of millions of people at risk for CKD or with a diagnosis of CKD via their service centers around the country. Partnering with them represents an attractive opportunity for the Network in terms of patient recruitment.

Contract Research Organizations (CROs) and Biotech Researchers are turning to RWD and RWE to support clinical trial design, observational studies, and generate new treatment approaches. The NKF Patient Network will offer the data to assist with these goals. We will engage with CROs and biotech companies that are interested in being either customers or partners of the Network.

Federal Agencies Federal agencies may engage with the Network either as funders (e.g., National Institute of Health, Patient-Centered Outcomes Research Institute, etc.) and/or members of the Governance committees to provide guidance on policy making and monitoring. As the largest, most comprehensive and longstanding non-profit health organization dedicated to the awareness, prevention, and treatment of kidney disease, NKF is well-positioned in nurturing these relationships.

Other Registries   Patient registries are utilized worldwide to collect data of patients with kidney disease due to different causes. Examples are the Nephrotic Syndrome Study Network (NEPTUNE), RADAR, CureGN, NURTuRE, and the ADPKD registry [9–13]. We aim to promote other registries on our Portal and create an international consortium for the recruitment of patients with kidney disease in clinical trials.

NKF Patient Network—Governance

The NKF Patient Network is expected to be operational for many years to come. It will be overseen by NKF but implemented and maintained with robust governance that involves the main stakeholders and a group of external experts from multiple disciplines (Fig. 5.3). The NKF will have contractual agreements with two entities that play an important role in the governance structure: the technology vendor, Pulse, and the Data Coordinating Center (DCC). Pulse is in charge of the data storage, cleaning, and security; data access to partners; extraction of datasets upon DCC request; and implementation of technology enhancements. The DCC will define datasets for research and collaborate with investigators in conducting statistical analyses for all approved research proposals that will lead to scientific publications, presentations, and abstracts.

The NKF also oversees the Steering Committee (SC) whose role is to assess the progress in achieving the Network objectives; recommend ongoing refinements of the patient portal and patient engagement strategy; and oversee the operations of the NKF Patient Network governance committees. Pharma sponsors and researchers were assigned an equal number of seats on this committee, because the project was made possible by their foundational support (Fig. 5.3). As the Network grows and evolves, the composition of the SC may change to reflect the recruitment of new partners.

The other governance committees are all working committees which recommend to the SC suggestions for efficient operations growth and innovations. The inclusion of all stakeholders in relevant committees helps to optimize authentic participation. Current working committees include:

- The Data Input and Integration Committee, which has significant representation of sponsors and academia that together defined the data dictionary (Fig. 5.2). The responsibilities of this committee are to lead the project in data access strategy development; provide feedback on major data integration plans between the various health care organizations, patient portal, and other data sources; and develop and approve changes to the data dictionary (completed Fall 2019).
- The Data Use and Publications Committee, which must approve all scientific publications, presentations, and abstracts using the NKF Patient Network data.

Pharma sponsor representatives were intentionally excluded from this committee to avoid conflict of interests. Other responsibilities of the committee are to oversee and update the Data Use and Publications policy (completed Fall 2019) and work with SC to select and ultimately oversee the DCC when sufficient data will be available for analysis (anticipated Fall 2021).

- The Technology Committee, which collaborates with Pulse to oversee the development and functionality of the platform, specifically content management between the NKF website and the platform. It also advises on potential tech innovations or additional features to improve patient engagement. Membership on this committee is restricted to constituents who have technical expertise.
- The Finance Committee, run by NKF representatives, which oversees the financial management, including fundraising and contracts of the project.

The main challenge we anticipate in running the operations of the Network is to keep the interest and the voice of patients central to the mission of the Network. To this end, patient representatives sit on all committees (except the Finance Committee that is internal to NKF) and together form the Patient Advisory Group. Patients were selected among the patient advocates who previously worked with NKF on other initiatives, proved to be excellent communicators, and showed selfless passion in serving the scientific community. Patients were also selected to represent the four personas that we predict will interact with the Network. The main responsibility of the Patient Advisory Group is to bring the patient perspective to the attention of the SC through its appointed constituents on the committee. We also envision that this will be a means to educate and engage patients and encourage their participation into larger roles within the Network.

All Committees perform their functions primarily via email with twice a year conference calls over a two-year term. To execute their functions, Governance Committee members receive updates on any progress in the project, are engaged with the Network activities, and have access to resources that will allow them to

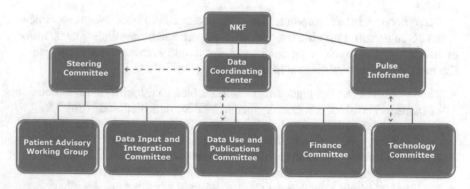

Fig. 5.3 NKF Patient Network Governance Structure. Orange lines represent contractual agreements; dotted lines represent collaborative efforts

take informed decisions. A subcommittee within the SC will evaluate the overall governance operations and the involvement of patients and HCPs in the governance committees and in research. The subcommittee will be composed of the chair of the SC, NKF executives, patient, and academia constituents. Pharma representatives will be excluded from this subcommittee because of the potential conflict of interest. NKF executives will evaluate separately the engagement with governance of sponsors and contractors (i.e., Pulse and DCC) and bring those findings to the subcommittee to review.

NKF Patient Network Model Will be Useful for Other National Registries

The NKF Patient Network is a unique example of multi-stakeholder collaboration and broadly engaged team science that unites efforts in the fight against kidney disease. Multiple stakeholders have been engaged in this project, including health care providers, pharmaceutical company sponsors, and a variety of others with interest in understanding, preventing, and treating CKD and its comorbidities. In the future, we hope that our model will be useful for other national registries that aim at accelerating research focused on patient outcomes, perceptions, priorities, and activities for other chronic diseases.

Acknowledgements The authors thank the NKF Patient Network partners (in alphabetical order): Geisinger, Pulse Infoframe, and Tufts Medical Center. The authors would also like to thank all the members of the governance committees (in alphabetical order): **Steering Committee:** Anne Barr, Brown and Toland; Lisa Bonebrake, Alport Syndrome Foundation; Kerry Cooper, AstraZeneca; Clarissa Diamantidis, Duke University School of Medicine; Barbara Gillespie, Labcorp Drug Development and University of North Carolina; Lesley Inker, Tufts Medical Center; Keren Ladin, Tufts University; Cari Maxwell, patient advocate; Amit Sharma, Bayer; Leslie Spry, Bryan Medical Center; Andre Stuerzenbecher, Bayer; Navdeep Tangri, University of Manitoba; Curtis Warfield, patient advocate. **Data Input And Integration Committee:** Shaun Bender, Boehringer Ingelheim; Kent Bressler, patient advocate; Kerri Cavanaugh, Vanderbilt Medical Center; Alex Chang, Geisinger; Samuel Fatoba, Bayer; Femida Gwadry-Sridhar, Pulse Infoframe; Lesley Inker, Tufts Medical Center; Sachin Paranjape, AstraZeneca; Michael Rocco, Wake Forest School of Medicine; Rakesh Singh, Bayer; Silvia Titan, Tufts Medical Center; Kerry Willis, National Kidney Foundation. **Data Use And Publications Committee:** Mary Baliker, patient advocate; Shoshana Ballew, Johns Hopkins; Lesley Inker, Tufts Medical Center; Nelson Kopyt, Lehigh Valley Health Network; Kristi Mitchell, Chief; Keith Norris, UCLA; Kerry Willis, National Kidney Foundation. **Finance Committee:** Stephanie Cogan, National Kidney Foundation; Petros Gregoriou, National Kidney Foundation; Anthony Gucciardo, National Kidney Foundation; Kerry Willis, National Kidney Foundation. **Technology Committee:** Anne Barr, Brown and Toland; Silvia Ferrè, National Kidney Foundation; Elizabeth Montgomery, National Kidney Foundation; Will Williams, National Kidney Foundation; Kerry Willis, National Kidney Foundation; Shanna Sutton, patient advocate. **Patient Advisory Working Group:** Mary Baliker, patient advocate; Luz Baqueiro, patient advocate; Aparna Baxi, patient advocate; Kent Bressler, patient advocate; Rachel Claudin, National Kidney Foundation; Kelli Collins, National Kidney Foundation; Derek Forfang, patient advocate; Cari Maxwell, patient advocate; Anthony Reed, patient advocate; Janine Reed, patient advocate, Alport Syndrome Foundation; Shanna Sutton, patient advocate; Curtis Warfield, patient advocate.

Funding Source Founding Sponsor: Bayer AG; Principal Sponsors: AstraZeneca, Boehringer Ingelheim, and Novartis.

References

1. KDIGO (2012) Clinical practice guideline for the evaluation and Management of Chronic Kidney Disease (2013). Office Journal of the International Society of Nephrology 3(1)
2. Levey AS, Coresh J (2012) Chronic kidney disease. Lancet 379(9811):165–180. https://doi.org/10.1016/S0140-6736(11)60178-5
3. Levey AS, Stevens LA, Schmid CH, Zhang YL, Castro AF 3rd, Feldman HI, Kusek JW, Eggers P, Van Lente F, Greene T, Coresh J, Ckd EPI (2009) A new equation to estimate glomerular filtration rate. Ann Intern Med 150(9):604–612. https://doi.org/10.7326/0003-4819-150-9-200905050-00006
4. Sarnak MJ, Amann K, Bangalore S, Cavalcante JL, Charytan DM, Craig JC, Gill JS, Hlatky MA, Jardine AG, Landmesser U, Newby LK, Herzog CA, Cheung M, Wheeler DC, Winkelmayer WC, Marwick TH, Conference P (2019) Chronic kidney disease and coronary artery disease: JACC state-of-the-art review. J Am Coll Cardiol 74(14):1823–1838. https://doi.org/10.1016/j.jacc.2019.08.1017
5. Annual Data Report. USRDS. https://www.usrds.org/annual-data-report/. Accessed 25 April 2020
6. Chronic Kidney Disease (CKD) Surveillance System. Centers for Disease Control and Prevention. https://nccd.cdc.gov/CKD/default.aspx. Accessed 27 April 2020
7. Plantinga LC, Tuot DS, Powe NR (2010) Awareness of chronic kidney disease among patients and providers. Adv Chronic Kidney Dis 17(3):225–236. https://doi.org/10.1053/j.ackd.2010.03.002
8. Chatzimanouil MKT, Wilkens L, Anders HJ (2019) Quantity and reporting quality of kidney research. J Am Soc Nephrol 30(1):13–22. https://doi.org/10.1681/ASN.2018050515
9. Kidney Research UK. https://kidneyresearchuk.org/. Accessed 25 April 2020
10. NEPHCURE Kidney International. https://nephcure.org/. Accessed 25 April 2020
11. Cure Glomerulonephropathy Network. CureGN. https://curegn.org/. Accessed 25 April 2020
12. PKD Foundation. https://pkdcure.org/. Accessed 25 April 2020
13. Rare Renal Information on rare kidney diseases. https://rarerenal.org/radar-registry/. Accessed 25 April 2020
14. Wagner EH, Austin BT, Davis C, Hindmarsh M, Schaefer J, Bonomi A (2001) Improving chronic illness care: translating evidence into action. Health Aff (Millwood) 20(6):64–78. https://doi.org/10.1377/hlthaff.20.6.64
15. Schmittdiel J, Bodenheimer T, Solomon NA, Gillies RR, Shortell SM (2005) Brief report: the prevalence and use of chronic disease registries in physician organizations. A national survey. J Gen Intern Med 20(9):855–858. https://doi.org/10.1111/j.1525-1497.2005.0171.x
16. Norris KC, Duru OK, Alicic RZ, Daratha KB, Nicholas SB, McPherson SM, Bell DS, Shen JI, Jones CR, Moin T, Waterman AD, Neumiller JJ, Vargas RB, Bui AAT, Mangione CM, Tuttle KR, investigators C-C (2019) Rationale and design of a multicenter chronic kidney disease (CKD) and at-risk for CKD electronic health records-based registry: CURE-CKD. BMC Nephrol 20 (1):416. doi:https://doi.org/10.1186/s12882-019-1558-9
17. Tuttle KR, Alicic RZ, Duru OK, Jones CR, Daratha KB, Nicholas SB, McPherson SM, Neumiller JJ, Bell DS, Mangione CM, Norris KC (2019) Clinical characteristics of and risk factors for chronic kidney disease among adults and children: an analysis of the CURE-CKD registry. JAMA Netw Open 2(12):e1918169. https://doi.org/10.1001/jamanetworkopen.2019.18169
18. Mendu ML, Ahmed S, Maron JK, Rao SK, Chaguturu SK, May MF, Mutter WP, Burdge KA, Steele DJR, Mount DB, Waikar SS, Weilburg JB, Sequist TD (2019) Development of an

electronic health record-based chronic kidney disease registry to promote population health management. BMC Nephrol 20(1):72. https://doi.org/10.1186/s12882-019-1260-y

19. CMS Blue Button 2.0. https://bluebutton.cms.gov/. Accessed 25 April 2020
20. National Institute of Diabetes and Digestive and Kidney Diseases. https://www.niddk.nih.gov/. Accessed 26 April 2020
21. Kidneys and Your Health. National Kidney Foundation. https://www.kidney.org/phi/form?version=health. Accessed 25 April 2020

Chapter 6
Broadly Engaged Team Science Comes to Life in a Design Lab

Marisha E. Palm, Harry P. Selker, Theodora Cohen, Kenneth I. Kaitin, Kay Larholt, Mark Trusheim, and Gigi Hirsch

Abstract The objective of broadly engaged team science is to bring a diverse group of stakeholders into a project early and continue to include their expertise throughout to inform and propel projects to successful and impactful outcomes. Broadly engaged team science goes beyond standard definitions of stakeholder engagement, bringing experts from relevant fields together with patients and members of the public not simply to engage or provide feedback, but to work together as a transdisciplinary team, where traditional boundaries are transcended. In this chapter we discuss the aspects of broadly engaged team science that are being developed and applied to advance biomedical research using a systems-level approach. We highlight the Design Lab, a successful context and process for getting wide-ranging stakeholder input and ensuring that stakeholder needs provide a framework for health care researchers and developers. We describe the Design Lab's methodology, its evolution, and where it has provided value.

Keywords Design Lab · NEWDIGS · biomedical value chain · FoCUS Consortium · LEAPS project

M. E. Palm (✉) · H. P. Selker · T. Cohen
Institute for Clinical Research and Health Policy Studies, Tufts Medical Center, Boston, MA, USA

Tufts Clinical and Translational Science Institute, Boston, MA, USA
e-mail: mpalm@tuftsmedicalcenter.org

K. I. Kaitin
Tufts Center for the Study of Drug Development, Tufts University School of Medicine, Boston, MA, USA

K. Larholt · M. Trusheim · G. Hirsch
NEW Drug Development ParadIGmS, Massachusetts Institute of Technology, Boston, MA, USA

© The Author(s), under exclusive license to Springer Nature Switzerland AG 2022
D. Lerner et al. (eds.), *Broadly Engaged Team Science in Clinical and Translational Research*, https://doi.org/10.1007/978-3-030-83028-1_6

The objective of broadly engaged team science is to bring a diverse group of stakeholders into a project early and continue to include their expertise throughout to inform and propel projects to successful and impactful outcomes. Broadly engaged team science goes beyond standard definitions of stakeholder engagement, bringing experts from relevant fields together with patients and members of the public not simply to engage or provide feedback, but to work together as a transdisciplinary team, where traditional boundaries are transcended. In this chapter we discuss the aspects of broadly engaged team science that are being developed and applied to advance biomedical research using a systems-level approach. We highlight the Design Lab, a successful context and process for getting wide-ranging stakeholder input and ensuring that stakeholder needs provide a framework for health care researchers and developers. We describe the Design Lab's methodology, its evolution, and where it has provided value.

The concept of the Design Lab was originally developed by collaborators within the **NEW** Drug **D**evelopment Parad**IG**m**S** (NEWDIGS) group at Massachusetts Institute of Technology (MIT). Their aim was to create a safe haven where stakeholders could collaborate and work toward sustainable, patient-centered biomedical innovation at a systems-level, with a focus on the biopharmaceutical and health care industries. Biomedical innovation involves a wide array of stakeholders, including manufacturers, biopharmaceutical companies, regulators, public health officials, public and private payers, provider systems, purchasers, clinicians, academic researchers, patients, patient advocates, and caregivers. While these groups often recognize the benefits of working together, collaboration can be supported by an external safe haven environment with a neutral intermediary to catalyze innovative solutions to difficult problems. Design Labs were developed to support a form of broadly engaged team science that brings multi-stakeholder groups together to brainstorm and innovate with the aim of accelerating biomedical innovation that is patient-centered and also works for all stakeholders.

Design Lab Methodology

Design Labs are highly interactive, hands-on working sessions that provide a pre-competitive environment, bringing potentially competing companies or individuals together to work toward a common goal [1]. Projects selected to be part of a Design Lab must have at least three different stakeholders with interest in the work. In addition, the atmosphere of the Design Lab must be carefully structured to support expansive engagement among stakeholders in order to address issues that are relevant across the biomedical value chain, including priority setting, research and development, regulatory approval, and access and use in clinical care. For these reasons, the essential elements of a Design Lab are that it: (1) is by invitation only, and invitation is guided by stakeholder mapping; (2) follows a case-based approach, with real life issues of relevance to biomedical research discussed; (3) fosters candid discussions by creating a safe haven.

When planning a Design Lab, invitations are sent to a carefully selected group of stakeholders. The stakeholder mapping process was developed by the NEWDIGS team and involves systematic consideration of stakeholders within relevant jurisdictions who represent key decision-makers, critical domains of expertise, and agents from across the innovation diffusion continuum (i.e., from early adopters to laggards). Critical stakeholder perspectives for the planned case discussions are identified by the NEWDIGS working team that develops the case presentation. Stakeholders who provide different standpoints and expertise are identified through outreach within the broad NEWDIGS community. The intentional inclusion of a variety of relevant stakeholders and therefore a variety of perspectives is one of the most important elements of the Design Lab.

NEWDIGS developed and then refined a set of guiding principles for the Design Labs to support the integrity and power of a safe haven culture. For example, the host of the Design Lab serves as a neutral intermediary for issues that may arise around competition and conflicts of interest and as the "steward" of the collaborative design process. The sessions operate under Chatham House Rules, whereby ideas may be shared following the sessions, but without attribution to specific individuals or organizations [2]. In addition, no binding decisions are made in a Design Lab session. This guiding principle was established to differentiate Design Labs from formal scientific advice sessions in the industry and to foster candid dialogue in the room, particularly with regulators and payers.

A range of topics have been tackled using the Design Lab methodology. These topics are often focused on system-wide challenges in health care. For example, a series of Design Labs focused on developing more flexible, evidence-driven approaches to paying for high cost, potentially curative new gene therapies that ensure access for patients, affordability for payers, and sustainability for developers. Another series focused on advancing from the traditional one-size-fits-all model of regulatory approval to a staged rollout to specific sub-populations informed by ongoing generation of real-world evidence. At Tufts, Design Labs have focused on innovative clinical trial designs that could improve trial efficiency and effectiveness by considering the information needs of a variety of stakeholders.

Design Lab Evolution 2010–2020

NEWDIGS began in 2010 and developed the concept of the Design Lab as a core element of its work in 2011. At that time, there was a growing awareness of the importance of multi-stakeholder collaboration as an approach to solving system challenges in the biopharmaceutical industry. Since the launch of MIT NEWDIGS Design Labs, the methods and tools that enable system-level innovation have developed and evolved, helping to advance our collective understanding of how to enable productivity and impact in these complex collaborative environments [3].

In 2016, Tufts Institute for Clinical Research and Health Policy Studies and Tufts Clinical and Translational Science Institute (hereafter jointly referred to as Tufts) began collaborating with MIT NEWDIGS to run Design Labs as part of their work with the Johns Hopkins University-Tufts Trial Innovation Center (JHU-Tufts TIC). The JHU-Tufts TIC is part of the Trial Innovation Network, a collaborative national network that focuses on operational innovation, with the aim of addressing road-blocks in clinical research and accelerating the translation of biomedical research. The methods used in the Design Lab, and the attention placed on bringing diverse stakeholders together, makes the Design Lab an ideal environment for developing innovative system-level solutions to improve the design, conduct, and impact of clinical trials.

The NEWDIGs program originally developed Design Labs to support health care industry collaboration. Tufts adapted the structure for use in designing and implementing National Institutes of Health and other federally-funded health care research. The framework provides support for investigators who are interested in innovations in clinical effectiveness research [e.g. 4–6]. Innovative clinical trial designs can work to address the effectiveness and safety gaps that are often present in standard clinical trials, providing a better understanding of how treatments will work in real-world settings. The Design Lab group discussion sessions hosted by Tufts and MIT NEWDIGs are structured to: consider case study stakeholders and what evidence they require; review the strengths and trade-offs of different study designs; and plan for any facilitators or challenges to clinical adoption. These sessions have supported health care researchers to develop better, more patient-centered study designs and consider plans for implementation and access. The pandemic has underscored some of the system-level challenges with clinical trials as well as an openness to innovative solutions [7].

MIT NEWDIGs has received requests to develop ways of supporting the dissemination and adoption of the Design Lab methodology for use within other parts of its organization using cross-functional teams. The group is now exploring ways to scale the processes and associated toolkit as a means of enhancing capacity for collaborative innovation beyond NEWDIGS and across the biomedical and health-care ecosystem. The work being done as part of the JHU-Tufts TIC is expanding the adoption of the Design Lab methodology, with the NEWDIGS team acting as consultants and supporting use of the methodology within a national network.

Design Lab Value

NEWDIG's Design Labs have worked to address system-level innovations and provided significant value in a number of important areas. Design Labs have brought multi-stakeholder, transdisciplinary teams together to focus on drug development and adaptive pharmaceutical product licensing, mapping stakeholders in a deliberate and inclusive way [8].

The output of each Design Lab is different, according to the questions being considered and the resulting brainstorm and discussion about solutions and next steps. Design Labs have met their objective of accelerating change in biomedicine;

they have led to changes in regulation that have been successfully piloted across Europe [9–13] and provided "precision financing" models for durable and potentially curative cell and gene therapies [14, 15]. Beyond these outputs, Design Labs have connected silos, built strong multi-stakeholder working relationships between groups that had not worked together before, encouraged participants to think more broadly and consider a wider variety of stakeholder needs, and provided an expansive strategic vision for sustainable, patient-centered innovation to inform future work [8].

The NEWDIGs-led Financing and Reimbursement of Cures in the US (FoCUS) Consortium is a collaborative project to improve financing models for durable, potentially curative therapies for cancers and genetic disorders [14–17]. Multi-stakeholder events, conferences and workshops were held to help people look at challenges to financing new cell and gene therapies and plan solutions. The Consortium concentrated on issues of patient access, affordability, and sustainability, and developed FoCUS Paying for Cures toolkit [18]. This toolkit is a collection of methodologies and tools that emphasize the need to tailor payment mechanisms to align with product and disease characteristics, as well as patient and family risks and financial challenges. It has enabled identification of seven different models with high potential to support financing solutions for durable, potentially curative therapies with large upfront costs and benefits that accrue over time.

The goal of the Learning Ecosystems Accelerator for Patient-centered, Sustainable innovation (LEAPS) project is to design and pilot a learning ecosystem that "gets the right treatment to the right patient at the right time." Success is defined as better clinical outcomes for patients and reducing waste and inefficiency across the system. The LEAPS collaborator community has worked together over a series of Design Labs to: create a shared vision for the learning ecosystem; select a target disease (Rheumatoid Arthritis, RA) for prototyping; and develop a "Learning Lifecycle Design Framework" to guide and coordinate development of the technologies, processes, policies, and incentives important for the success and sustainability of the learning ecosystem. Like a learning health care system, a learning ecosystem has embedded knowledge generation processes and supports improvement toward better patient outcomes. The LEAPS Design Labs have provided the environment and structure for stakeholders to prototype components of this learning system to optimize drug therapy regimens for RA. They have also provided a valuable way of engaging real world partners who will collaborate on implementation and scaling, as well as translation to other diseases that could benefit from improved evidence generation.

In the Design Labs that Tufts has hosted, innovative approaches to clinical effectiveness in multi-site trials are discussed, and the trial designs are built with all of the stakeholders' needs in mind. One of the Tufts Design Labs focused on the repurposing of an approved drug in a condition where there is currently a lack of optimal care and a high rate of mortality. The Design Lab focused on the evidence required by different stakeholders to enable accelerated approval and adoption and looked at how best to generate that evidence. Some of the generalizable discussion points were that there is a growing demand for a demonstration of effectiveness (i.e., how well a product or therapeutic works in a real-world setting), and that the outcomes of effectiveness that matter may be different for different stakeholders (e.g., payers, prescribers, and patients). The Design Lab created a space for investigators to think beyond the science of biomedicine and allowed them to build a more fully developed plan for approvals, access, and use of the treatment in clinical care.

Design Lab Methods and Tools Continue to Evolve

We have seen broadly engaged team science come to life in Design Labs. These collaborative, safe haven environments bring diverse stakeholders together to tackle important scientific questions and help modernize biomedical and health care systems so they can function more effectively. In addition, the methodology of Design Labs supports mapping stakeholder needs and thinking about scientific evidence generation in the context of these needs. Design Lab methods and tools continue to evolve through their ongoing application to new challenges and opportunities.

References

1. Baird L, Hirsch G (2013) Adaptive licensing: creating a safe haven for discussions. Scrip Regulatory Affairs:10–11
2. Chatham House Rule. Chatham House. https://www.chathamhouse.org/chatham-house-rule
3. Papadaki M, Hirsch G (2013) Curing Consortium Fatigue. Science Translational Medicine 5(200):200fs235. https://doi.org/10.1126/scitranslmed.3006903
4. Selker HP, Oye KA, Eichler HG, Stockbridge NL, Mehta CR, Kaitin KI, McElwee NE, Honig PK, Erban JK, D'Agostino RB (2014) A proposal for integrated efficacy-to-effectiveness (E2E) clinical trials. Clin Pharmacol Ther 95(2):147–153. https://doi.org/10.1038/clpt.2013.177
5. Selker HP, Eichler HG, Stockbridge NL, McElwee NE, Dere WH, Cohen T, Erban JK, Seyfert-Margolis VL, Honig PK, Kaitin KI, Oye KA, D'Agostino RB (2019) Efficacy and effectiveness too trials: clinical trial designs to generate evidence on efficacy and on effectiveness in wide practice. Clin Pharmacol Ther 105(4):857–866. https://doi.org/10.1002/cpt.1347
6. Kravitz RL, Duan N, eds, and the DEcIDE Methods Center N-of-1 Guidance Panel (Duan N, Eslick I, Gabler NB, Kaplan HC, Kravitz RL, Larson EB, Pace WD, Schmid CH, Sim I, Vohra S). Design and Implementation of N-of-1 Trials: A User's Guide. AHRQ Publication No. 13(14)-EHC122-EF. Rockville, MD: Agency for Healthcare Research and Quality; January 2014
7. Innovation to Respond to COVID-19: FDA and Partners Aim to Capture Real-World Data to Identify Potential Treatments for Further Study (2021). https://www.fda.gov/emergency-preparedness-and-response/coronavirus-disease-2019-covid-19/innovation-respond-covid-19
8. Hirsch G (2019) Leaping together toward sustainable, patient-centered innovation: the value of a multistakeholder safe haven for accelerating system change. Clin Pharmacol Ther 105(4):798–801. https://doi.org/10.1002/cpt.1237
9. Eichler HG, Oye K, Baird LG, Abadie E, Brown J, Drum CL, Ferguson J, Garner S, Honig P, Hukkelhoven M, Lim JC, Lim R, Lumpkin MM, Neil G, O'Rourke B, Pezalla E, Shoda D, Seyfert-Margolis V, Sigal EV, Sobotka J, Tan D, Unger TF, Hirsch G (2012) Adaptive licens-

ing: taking the next step in the evolution of drug approval. Clin Pharmacol Ther 91(3):426–437. https://doi.org/10.1038/clpt.2011.345

10. Baird L, Teagarden R, Unger T, Hirsch G (2013) New medicines eight years faster to patients: blazing a new trail in drug development with adaptive licensing. Scrip Regulatory Affairs

11. Eichler HG, Baird LG, Barker R, Bloechl-Daum B, Borlum-Kristensen F, Brown J, Chua R, Del Signore S, Dugan U, Ferguson J, Garner S, Goettsch W, Haigh J, Honig P, Hoos A, Huckle P, Kondo T, Le Cam Y, Leufkens H, Lim R, Longson C, Lumpkin M, Maraganore J, O'Rourke B, Oye K, Pezalla E, Pignatti F, Raine J, Rasi G, Salmonson T, Samaha D, Schneeweiss S, Siviero PD, Skinner M, Teagarden JR, Tominaga T, Trusheim MR, Tunis S, Unger TF, Vamvakas S, Hirsch G (2015) From adaptive licensing to adaptive pathways: delivering a flexible life-span approach to bring new drugs to patients. Clin Pharmacol Ther 97(3):234–246. https://doi.org/10.1002/cpt.59

12. Schulthess D, Baird LG, Trusheim M, Unger TF, Lumpkin M, Hoos A, Garner S, Gavin P, Goldman M, Seigneuret N, Chlebus M, Van Baelen K, Bergstrom R, Hirsch G (2016) Medicines adaptive pathways to patients (MAPPs): a story of international collaboration leading to implementation. Ther Innov Regul Sci 50(3):347–354. https://doi.org/10.1177/2168479015618697

13. Blackburn S (2017) Adaptive pathways are creating win-win scenarios for patients and pharma. AccessPoint, QuintilesIMS Real-World Insights 7

14. Precision Financing Solutions for Durable/Potentially Curative Therapies (2019) MIT NEWDIGS White Paper

15. Tools for Implementation of Precision Financing Solutions Within Medicaid Plans Part 1 (2019) MIT NEWDIGS White Paper

16. Learning Ecosystems Accelerator for Patient-centered, Sustainable Innovation Part 2 (2020) MIT NEWDIGS Research Brief

17. Learning Ecosystems Accelerator for Patient-centered, Sustainable Innovation (2020) MIT NEWDIGS Research Brief

18. FoCUS Project at MIT: Paying for Cures Toolkit (2021). https://payingforcures.mit.edu/toolkit/

Chapter 7
Tufts Center for the Study of Drug Development Employs Broadly Engaged Team Science to Explore the Challenges of Pharmaceutical Research and Development

Kenneth I. Kaitin and Kenneth Getz

Abstract Tufts Center for the Study of Drug Development (CSDD) is a multidisciplinary research center at Tufts University School of Medicine. Tufts CSDD conducts research to explore the economic, regulatory, scientific, and political factors that affect the development and approval of new pharmaceutical products. In many of its studies, Tufts CSDD critically relies on broadly engaged team science to capture the views of and incorporate data provided by its varied stakeholders. These stakeholders include research-based pharmaceutical companies, contract service providers, clinical investigators, patient advocacy groups, technology companies, investors, government regulators, and the United States (US) Department of Defense. Their input is used to help design studies, create surveys, provide data, interpret results, and disseminate findings.

Keywords Tufts Center for the Study of Drug Development (CSDD) · Drug development · Pharmaceutical R&D · Cost of drug development · Drug development process

Tufts Center for the Study of Drug Development (CSDD) is a multidisciplinary academic research center focused on the economic, regulatory, scientific, and political factors that affect biomedical innovation [1]. For over four decades[1] Tufts CSDD

---

[1] The Center for the Study of Drug Development was founded in 1976 at the University of Rochester in Rochester, NY, by visionary physician Dr. Louis Lasagna. The group moved to Tufts University in 1984.

K. I. Kaitin (✉) · K. Getz
Tufts Center for the Study of Drug Development, Tufts University School of Medicine, Boston, MA, USA
e-mail: kenneth.kaitin@tufts.edu

© The Author(s), under exclusive license to Springer Nature Switzerland AG 2022
D. Lerner et al. (eds.), *Broadly Engaged Team Science in Clinical and Translational Research*, https://doi.org/10.1007/978-3-030-83028-1_7

55

has provided widely cited benchmarks on the time, cost, and risk of new drug development, examined the impact of regulatory initiatives to stimulate and speed the drug development process, and reported on efforts to boost research and development (R&D) efficiency and productivity. Tufts CSDD also offers professional development courses and hosts workshops and public forums on a wide range of drug development issues. The mission of Tufts CSDD is to provide data-driven analysis, strategic insight, and educational programming to improve the development and regulatory process for new pharmaceutical products.

The Current Drug Development Landscape

The drug development enterprise is often referred to as an "ecosystem," reflecting the numerous individuals and organizations involved in successfully bringing a new medicine to market. These include academic scientists, clinical investigators, government funding agencies, venture financing, small pharmaceutical companies, start-ups, large multinational firms, non-profit organizations, patient advocacy groups, payers, technology companies, and contract service providers. Tufts CSDD works closely with many of these stakeholders to better understand drug development challenges and to assess efforts to improve the development process.

The primary challenge for drug developers today is the stubbornly risky, time-consuming, and expensive process by which new medicines are developed and brought to market. Based on analyses conducted by Tufts CSDD, the average capitalized cost to bring one new pharmaceutical product to market, including the cost of failures, is $2.6 billion [2]. This figure represents a 145% increase over Tufts CSDD's previous cost estimate (in constant dollars) reported in 2003. The high cost of drug development reflects, in part, the difficulty in developing products for chronic and complex indications (for example, neurologic and immunologic diseases), the challenge of recruiting and retaining subjects for clinical trials, increasing protocol complexity, and late-stage failures in the drug development process.

Tufts CSDD data indicate that the average time to bring a pharmaceutical product to market, from synthesis to marketing approval, is about 15 years, approximately eight of which is spent in the clinical testing and regulatory approval phases of development. Moreover, the likelihood of clinical success is only 11.8%, meaning that few candidates that begin clinical testing will eventually make it to the market. Of course, these numbers mask considerable variability across different therapeutic areas. For example, the time from the start of clinical testing to submission of a new drug application (NDA) or biologics licensing application (BLA) to the US. Food and Drug Administration (FDA) ranges from 6.3 years for anti-infective drugs to 9.4 years for drugs to treat gastrointestinal diseases and disorders. Similarly, overall clinical approval success rates (i.e., the likelihood that a candidate starting clinical testing will eventually be approved for marketing) ranges from 23.9% for systemic anti-infectives to 3.7% for cardiovascular drugs [3].

Tufts CSDD's Multi-Stakeholder Working Groups and Engaged Team Science

To understand and report on the intricacies and complexities of the drug development process, one must rely on the input of those individuals and organizations on the frontline of pharmaceutical R&D, including academic researchers, clinical investigators, industry drug developers, contract service and technology providers, and government regulators and policymakers. By mining the perspectives of these stakeholders, and by obtaining proprietary and non-proprietary development metrics from research-based organizations, Tufts CSDD is able to create a robust body of qualitative and quantitative data that serves as the basis for many of its research studies.

Tufts CSDD regularly employs multi-stakeholder working groups to tap into the well of stakeholder knowledge and experience and address important drug development issues [4]. These working groups take advantage of Tufts CSDD's worldwide reputation for scholarly analyses and its position as a neutral forum for the exchange of ideas, data, and solutions. Working group projects typically result in a comprehensive, data-driven report, which is then made available to a broad audience as a Tufts CSDD White Paper (available on our website) or a publication in a peer-reviewed or trade journal. In recent years, Tufts CSDD has conducted multi stakeholder working groups with pharmaceutical companies, investigative sites, patient advocacy groups, the US. Department of Defense, contract research organizations, and technology providers.

The typical workflow for a multi-stakeholder working group is as follows:

- Tufts CSDD, along with advisors, defines an appropriate research project to address a timely and important drug development issue.
- A notice, which includes the goals and objectives of the new working group, is posted on our website and is publicized in a press release. In some cases, specific participants are identified and contacted directly. In other cases, a general sign-up link is provided. There is also a general outreach to Tufts CSDD contacts and relevant organizations. A typical working group has participants representing 10–30 individual organizations, depending on the topic and the types of organizations engaged.
- An introductory in-person meeting is held at Tufts CSDD offices with all participants in the working group. At this meeting, after initial introductions, Tufts CSDD's lead investigator describes the premise and scope of the project and presents any preliminary or relevant prior research. The participants then have the opportunity to share experiences and express views on the project. A major goal of this meeting is to contribute to the formulation of a survey instrument, which will capture the data critical for the project analysis.
- Following the introductory meeting, Tufts CSDD finalizes the survey instrument and circulates it to the relevant parties for completion. Tufts CSDD project managers follow-up as needed to answer questions and prompt participants to complete the survey.

- Once the completed surveys are returned, Tufts CSDD analyzes the data and prepares a preliminary slide deck, containing findings and interpretations, to present to the working group participants.
- A second in-person meeting is held at Tufts CSDD offices with all participants to present the preliminary analysis and interpretations. At this meeting, participants are asked to reflect on the findings and consider if any additional analyses or interpretations are warranted.
- Following the second meeting, Tufts CSDD researchers finalize the analysis, prepare the report, and either submit a manuscript for peer-review publication or present the information as a white paper available on Tufts CSDD's website. Typically, analyses from these projects are also used in the preparation of a *Tufts CSDD Impact Report*, which is a bi-monthly subscription-based publication highlighting recently conducted original research [5].

The typical timeline from project concept to completion of final report is 6 to 9 months.

Specific Examples of Tufts CSDD Multi-Stakeholder Working Groups

"Examining Clinical Protocol Complexity in Drug Development"

Over the past 15 years, Tufts CSDD researchers have conducted approximately 40 multi-stakeholder working group studies looking at protocol design practices and their impact on drug development speed, cost, and efficiency. These particular working group studies usually engage between 20 and 30 major and mid-sized pharmaceutical and biotechnology companies, as well as contract service providers. The results of these working group studies have demonstrated that more complex protocols (e.g., number of endpoints, procedures, eligibility criteria, planned patient visits) are associated with poor clinical trial performance (e.g., longer cycle times, lower recruitment and retention rates, increased amendments). Study results have been published extensively in peer-reviewed and trade journals, book chapters, and in *Tufts CSDD Impact Reports* [6–9].

"Evaluating Barriers to the Development of New Treatments for Lupus"

Although lupus affects more than 5 million people globally and the prevalence of the disease is increasing, only one treatment has received approval and more than 30 others have failed during development over the past 60 years. Tufts CSDD, in collaboration with the Lupus Foundation of America (LFA), brought together a working group of companies, patients, and international lupus experts to examine barriers to the development of new lupus treatments. Through interviews and surveys, the working group found that the heterogeneity of lupus and the lack of a clear disease definition limit drug development progress. The results of the study have been published in a peer-review journal and as a *Tufts CSDD White Paper* [10, 11]. Notably, the study has informed a new consortium focusing on building disease definition consensus among practitioners, payers, and regulatory agencies [12].

"Assessing Pharma Industry's Adoption of Machine Learning and Artificial Intelligence"

Digital disruption is occurring throughout all areas of drug development. This working group gathered data on industry preparedness to leverage the use of machine learning and artificial intelligence to support clinical research planning and activity. Eight pharmaceutical companies participated in the development of an online survey that gathered responses from several hundred distinct organizations. The results indicate that a large percentage of companies are piloting the use of machine learning primarily to support biomarker identification, pharmacovigilance, patient identification, and real-world evidence evaluation. The study findings have been published in a peer-reviewed journal and in a *Tufts CSDD Impact Report* [13, 14]. They were also presented by Tufts CSDD at an expert hearing on artificial intelligence, organized by the US. Government Accountability Office (GAO) and the National Academy of Medicine (NAM), the proceedings of which were published in December 2019 [15].

Challenges and Limitations of Tufts CSDD's Multi-Stakeholder Working Groups and the Engaged Team Science Approach

There are several challenges and limitations inherent in the multi-stakeholder working group model. Following is a summary of these challenges and a description of Tufts CSDD's approach to managing them:

- *How do you make sure you are including the right and appropriate number of organizations in the working group?* At the outset of every new project, it is critical to clearly and concisely articulate the question being asked in the research. That helps with the identification of appropriate stakeholders for the project. For example, a study of how a new technology, such as machine learning, is affecting the drug development process, may benefit by including in the working group both research-based pharmaceutical firms that are using the technology, as well as those technology companies with expertise in that area. In general, every effort is made to encourage relevant organizations to participate in working groups. Sometimes that requires contacting those organizations directly to encourage their participation. There is typically no cap on the number of organizations that may participate. However, there are occasions when it is not possible to get a particularly important company to participate. In those cases, the project simply moves forward without their participation.

- *How do you get organizations that are normally competitors to work together on a project?* Despite the competitive nature of the biopharmaceutical and affiliated (e.g., contract service providers) industries, Tufts CSDD has found that they are joined by a common goal of improving the efficiency and productivity of the drug development process. Many of these companies are familiar with the scholarly and objective analyses and reports produced by Tufts CSDD, and they appreciate the opportunity to work together with colleagues in a neutral venue to engage in an academic, data-driven research program, with the goal of generating fact-based insights into improving R&D performance.
- *How do you maintain the confidentiality of proprietary data?* Many of Tufts CSDD's multi-stakeholder projects entail the collection of highly sensitive, proprietary data from research-based drug companies or other organizations. In most cases, these types of data are not shared outside of the organization. Nonetheless, companies typically are willing to share the information with Tufts CSDD for two reasons: (1) Tufts CSDD maintains a strict policy of never divulging proprietary data of any kind. These data may include, for example, information on management practices, drug development benchmarks, or R&D strategy. All Tufts CSDD analyses included in publications or public presentations are based on aggregate analyses only. (2) Tufts CSDD has a worldwide reputation for scholarly, objective, and influential analyses, spanning four and a half decades. Stakeholders are confident that their participation in a Tufts CSDD working group will result in a positive and meaningful research experience.
- *How do you accommodate fundamental differences among stakeholders from different types of organizations and get them to collaborate?* As mentioned above, the drug development enterprise is often thought of as an ecosystem. Different stakeholders are typically aware of and are used to working with other types of organizations. For example, many pharmaceutical companies work closely with contract research organizations, who provide clinical trial services. Tufts CSDD has not run into a situation where working group participants were unable to collaborate or where fundamental differences preluded the ability to produce useful analyses. To the contrary, most participants value and enjoy the opportunity to work together with colleagues from different organizations to achieve a common research goal.
- *How does Tufts CSDD ensure that it maintains objectivity and neutrality in its analysis and interpretation of results?* Tufts CSDD has a worldwide reputation for scholarly data-driven research. Tufts CSDD understands the importance of maintaining its objectivity and neutrality in its analysis and interpretation of research findings. To achieve this, databases are created, managed, and analyzed

by Tufts CSDD faculty and staff only. Moreover, most working groups result in manuscripts that are submitted to peer-reviewed journals, where study rationale, methodology, analysis, and interpretation are vetted to ensure appropriateness and lack of bias.

- *Is the multi-stakeholder working group model appropriate for all Tufts CSDD research projects?* The simple answer is, No. For some Tufts CSDD research projects, the multi-stakeholder working group model may be deemed inappropriate, unnecessary, or not feasible. Examples include the following: (1) Tufts CSDD regularly conducts economic evaluations of the cost of new drug development [16]. These studies, which determine the total capitalized cost to bring a new pharmaceutical product to market, generate enormous interest and debate within industrial, regulatory, and policy circles worldwide. Due to the politically sensitive nature of the topic and the use of highly proprietary company data on development costs, the study authors, comprised of three prominent economists from Tufts CSDD, Duke University, and University of Rochester, devise the study's methodology, collect and analyze the data, and interpret the results, without external input. (2) A second example is Tufts CSDD's assessment of FDA's implementation of Breakthrough Therapy Designation, a regulatory pathway to facilitate development and review of lifesaving drugs [17]. Because data for this study were available from public sources and through a memorandum of understanding Tufts CSDD has with the FDA – in which FDA annually provides Tufts CSDD with drug-specific regulatory milestone data – it was deemed unnecessary to convene a working group for this project. (3) As a final example, Tufts CSDD, and collaborator Shanghai Center for Drug Discovery and Development at Fudan University, conducted a study on recent reforms of the Chinese regulatory review process and their impact on access to important new medicines in China [18]. In this case, it was not considered feasible to formulate a working group that would include Chinese drug regulators and pharmaceutical companies.

Tufts CSDD's Multi-Stakeholder Working Group Approach Could Lead to New Drug Development Practices and Regulatory Standards

Tufts CSDD multi-stakeholder working groups represent a unique form of broadly engaged team science, leading to highly valuable assessments of, and solutions to, critical drug development challenges. In addition to generating important insights, these working groups provide a neutral forum for stakeholders from different organizations and industries to work together, learn from each other's experiences, and build trust.

Tufts CSDD, in its role as project manager and facilitator, encourages candor, openness, and a sense of common purpose among the participants. Post-working group feedback typically reflects a high level of participant enthusiasm and appreciation for having been integrally involved in the project. Importantly, participants also report that knowledge gained in the working group often result in actionable improvements in internal process and strategy.

New drug development is time-consuming, risky, and expensive. Tufts CSDD's multi-stakeholder working groups are a powerful methodological tool for capturing the unique complexities of the drug development process by tapping into the knowledge and insights of stakeholders involved in bringing new medicines to patients. In the future, more formal evaluation of the effectiveness of this approach could lead to new drug development practices and regulatory standards.

References

1. Tufts Center for the Study of Drug Development. https://csdd.tufts.edu/
2. DiMasi JA, Grabowski HG, Hansen RW (2016) Innovation in the pharmaceutical industry: new estimates of R&D costs. J Health Econ 47:20–33. https://doi.org/10.1016/j.jhealeco.2016.01.012
3. Cardiovascular drug approval rate in the U.S. fell as development time rose, according to the tufts center for the study of drug development (2017) Internet wire
4. Tufts CSDD Multi-Company Working Groups. https://csdd.tufts.edu/research-platforms-and-working-groups
5. Tufts CSDD Impact Reports. https://csdd.tufts.edu/impact-reports
6. Getz KA, Campo RA (2018) New benchmarks characterizing growth in protocol design complexity. Ther Innov Regul Sci 52(1):22–28. https://doi.org/10.1177/2168479017713039
7. Getz KA (2018) Transitions in the trial landscape: what will drive RCTs into the clinic? In Vivo 36(5):16–22
8. Getz KA, Kaitin KI (2015) The impact of bad protocols. Chapter 10. In: Re-engineering clinical trials: best practices for streamlining the development process. Shüler P, Buckley B (eds). London: Elsevier, Academic Press
9. Kaitin K (ed) (2018) Rising protocol design complexity is driving rapid growth in clinical trial data volume. Tufts Center for the Study of Drug Development Impact Report, vol 20, no 4. Tufts University
10. Peña Y, Tse K, Hanrahan LM, de Bruin A, Morand EF, Getz K (2020) Establishing consensus understanding of the barriers to drug development in lupus. Ther Innov Regul Sci 54(5):1159–1165. https://doi.org/10.1007/s43441-020-00134-2
11. Manzi S, Raymond S, Tse K, Pena Y, Anderson A, Arntsen K, Bae SC, Bruce I, Dorner T, Getz K, Hanrahan L, Kao A, Morand E, Rovin B, Schanberg LE, Von Feldt JM, Werth VP, Costenbader K (2019) Global consensus building and prioritisation of fundamental lupus challenges: the ALPHA project. Lupus Sci Med 6(1):e000342. https://doi.org/10.1136/lupus-2019-000342
12. Tse K, Hanrahan L, Pena Y, Getz K (2019) ALPHA project unites global lupus community on barriers to research, drug development, care and access. Tufts Center for the Study of Drug Development White Paper
13. International Lupus Community Reaches First-Ever Agreement on Barriers to Research, Drug Development, Care and Access (2019). https://www.lupus.org/news/international-lupus-community-reaches-firstever-agreement-on-barriers-to-research-drug#. Accessed May 5, 2020
14. Lamberti MJ, Wilkinson M, Donzanti BA, Wohlhieter GE, Parikh S, Wilkins RG, Getz K (2019) A study on the application and use of artificial intelligence to support drug development. Clin Ther 41(8):1414–1426. https://doi.org/10.1016/j.clinthera.2019.05.018

15. Kaitin K (ed) (2019) Adoption of artificial intelligence is high across drug development. Tufts Center for the Study of Drug Development Impact Report, vol 21, no 3. Tufts University
16. Artificial Intelligence in Health Care: Benefits and challenges of machine learning in drug development (2020) https://www.gao.gov/products/GAO-20-215SP
17. Kaitin K (ed) (2014) New breakthrough therapy designation program aims to cut clinical trial time. Tufts Center for the Study of Drug Development Impact Report, vol 15, no 1. Tufts University
18. Xu L, Gao H, Kaitin KI, Shao L (2018) Reforming China's drug regulatory system. Nat Rev Drug Discov 17(12):858–859. https://doi.org/10.1038/nrd.2018.150

Part II
Integrating Communities and Stakeholders into Broadly Engaged Team Science

Chapter 8
Social Movements and Stakeholder Engagement

Peter Levine

Abstract Social movements are among the most powerful sources of popular energy in our society. Scientists and health professionals should expect to see them burgeoning and shaping our understanding of medicine and population health, both for better and worse. This chapter describes challenges to the traditional way of thinking about social movements and explains why people who hold positions inside institutions—including medical researchers, clinicians, and health administrators—need to react to movements more analytically and more constructively. A model for assessing movements is presented. This model can help scientists and health professionals understand the strengths and weaknesses of social movements so they can better decide whether and how to engage with them.

Keywords Health-related social movements · Scale-Pluralism-Unity-Depth (SPUD) Framework · Broadly Engaged Team Science · Social movement dynamics

Social movements are among the most powerful sources of popular energy in our society. Scientists and health professionals should expect to see them burgeoning and shaping our understanding of medicine and population health, both for better and worse.

Some social movements focus explicitly on health issues, such as reproductive freedom and vaccination. The two most prominent social movements in the United States right now—those involving climate change and racial justice—do not focus on medicine or public health, per se, but they have pervasive implications for health care, for scientific and medical institutions, and for health policy. For instance, climate change affects population health; systemic racism is at the root of many health disparities.

Since the literature on social movements rarely distinguishes health-focused movements from other ones, I will draw implications from what is known about

P. Levine (✉)
Tisch College of Civic Life, Tufts University, Medford, MA, USA
e-mail: peter.levine@tufts.edu

© The Author(s), under exclusive license to Springer Nature
Switzerland AG 2022
D. Lerner et al. (eds.), *Broadly Engaged Team Science in Clinical and Translational Research*, https://doi.org/10.1007/978-3-030-83028-1_8

movements in general. However, medical scientists and other health professionals may reasonably focus on social movements that are explicitly concerned with health and on the impact of other movements on the health system and related professions.

As representatives of formal institutions, such as universities and hospitals—and as bearers of professional expertise—scientists and health professionals may begin with some skepticism about social movements. To evaluate a given movement, they may be tempted to ask only one question: whether its demands are consistent with a scientific consensus and their own institutions' agendas. Confronted by a movement against vaccination or against genetic research, they may respond defensively.

This response overlooks the full potential of social movements and misses the opportunity for partnerships that combine the empowerment of movements with the rigor of scientific disciplines. Forming such partnerships requires due appreciation of social movements and sophistication about how they work.

Such appreciation is especially important for proponents of broadly engaged team science, who are committed to engaging stakeholders [1]. Sometimes, stakeholders are not just individuals who may receive outreach from professionals but are participants in social movements who *demand* inclusion. All health professionals, and especially those who practice broadly engaged team science, need principles and skills for making the best of such demands.

How Science and Health Professionals Define "Engagement"

Scientists and stakeholders may call on at least three main approaches to guide engagement, and these differ according to who initiates the work. Much recent scholarship on engagement in health research is devoted to engagement of stakeholders that is initiated by researchers. A longer-standing set of frameworks addresses the needs of partnerships of communities and researchers who wish to work together on as-yet undefined research agendas. A third set, with more than a century of scholarship, speaks to engagement that is initiated by social movements.

The most recent of these approaches helps scientists to initiate the involvement of stakeholders in the planning, conduct, and dissemination of the researcher's existing agenda [2, 3]. This work defines a "stakeholder" in a health issue as any "individual or group who is responsible for or affected by health- and health care-related decisions that can be informed by research evidence." For them, one important set of stakeholders consists of "patients and the public," including "patient and consumer advocacy organizations." The same work defines "engagement" as "a bi-directional relationship between the stakeholder and researcher that results in informed decision-making about the selection, conduct, and use of research." They note that the first step of research is often "evidence prioritization," which means "establishing a vision and mission for research, identifying topics, setting priorities, and refining questions."

A longer-standing group of approaches helps partnerships of researchers and communities form new agendas for research and pursue them together [4]. In Community-Based Participatory Research and related frameworks, stakeholders are geographically defined community members who express an interest in research. Engagement is a power-sharing arrangement in which communities may have some or all control over research budgets, staffing decisions, and overall direction of the work.

Different frameworks are needed to help researchers respond competently to movements.

Health-Related Social Movements

A classic example of a health-related social movement developed around ACT UP (the AIDS Coalition to Unleash Power) and other groups focused on AIDS treatment in the 1980s. In a provocative article published in 1995, Steven Epstein argued that these activists did not merely advocate more research on HIV/AIDS or influence public beliefs about the epidemic. They also "constituted themselves as *credible participants in the process of knowledge construction*, thereby bringing about changes in the epistemic practices of biomedical research" [5, emphasis added].

AIDS activists used a wide range of tactics to change research agendas, funding, and attitudes toward gay men and others affected by the disease. Some of their methods, such as demonstrations and acts of civil disobedience, were highly public. Others were less visible. AIDS activists taught themselves science, identified and took positions on empirical and ethical controversies within the health disciplines, translated technical information from one scientific subfield to another, demanded new criteria for inclusion in clinical trials, and then helped to recruit subjects for these experiments, served on committees and advisory boards convened by conventional organizations like hospitals, universities and public agencies, and participated in formal conferences and negotiations about policy [5].

Many other social movements have also demanded changes in the agendas or practices of science [6, 7]. Our Bodies Ourselves and the anti-abortion movement have been powerful examples. Today, movements' causes range from environmental justice to anti-vaccination. Some focus on specific diseases or conditions, while others address the health of the entire planet. They use the full repertoire of social movement activism, including public demonstrations and disruptions like sit-ins, online expression, and support for political candidates, plus the same kinds of quiet, insider tactics that were important in the early AIDs movements.

Social movements have remained common or even grown while other forms of civic engagement have shrunk. In 1970, a substantial majority of American adults either attended a church weekly or belonged to a union, or both. Today, only about one-third are engaged in those traditional bulwarks of civil society [8]. On the other hand, the proportion of Americans who attended protests (an aspect of social movement participation) tripled between 1978 and 2007 [9]. As religious congregations and unions have waned, social movements have waxed, absorbing a higher proportion of our energy as a people.

McCarthy and Zald call a social movement "a set of opinions and beliefs in a population which represents preferences for changing some elements of the social structure and/or reward distribution of a society [10]." If this is an accurate depiction of movements, then when scientists and health professionals are confronted by a given movement, their questions become: Is this a legitimate group of stakeholders? Do their demands relate to the professionals' work? Do their opinions belong in the discussion? Do their protest activities indicate that they have a stake in the issue? Should we engage them?

In this framework, the AIDS treatment activists in Epstein's article could be understood as a group of patients, caregivers, and advocacy organizations who had bidirectional relationships with scientists and scientific organizations and helped identify topics, set priorities, and refine questions.

But did these activists constitute a "movement?" A Google Image Search of the phrase "social movement" returns photographs of masses of protesters in various public spaces, carrying signs with very similar slogans. That result suggests that a social movement is a label for *individuals* who hold *opinions* that they express in public *protests*. Similar definitions can also be found in older scholarly literature.

How Movements Work

I would like to challenge an approach to movements that treats them as groups of stakeholders with opinions whom institutions can choose to engage (or not).

First, the interaction between AIDS activists and scientists was not designed or initiated by professionals who worked inside institutions and who sought to promote engagement with selected patients and other stakeholders. To a significant extent, the interaction was forced on science by laypeople. Scientific institutions did not get to choose whether to engage.

Second, a "stakeholder" is often defined as someone with a "stake" or interest in a topic [11]. For instance, anyone with HIV has a stake in that issue. In contrast, social movement participants seek to demonstrate "worthiness," a right to a voice on the issue [12]. These are related but different ideas. You can be worthy to address an issue even if it doesn't affect you personally; perhaps you simply hold strong beliefs about it. A "stake" seems to be an empirical matter, something that an independent observer could assess. It is a matter of fact whether you are affected by an issue or not. Worthiness, on the other hand, is a moral claim. A person can earn worthiness by making sacrifices to participate in a movement.

Third, a movement is not just a population of potential stakeholders from which individuals can be selected to participate in organized, professionally-designed engagement processes or team science. Instead, a movement is an active entity with its own direction and force. Thus, movements often stretch typical definitions of "stakeholder groups."

Fourth, a movement does not simply represent one or a few opinions. Usually, it reflects diverse views on its own core issues and is a site of debate. Its agenda usually shifts and develops over time. Nor do people necessarily participate because they endorse the core positions of a movement. A frequent pattern is that people join protests because someone they trust invites them to participate; then, by protesting, they are convinced of the movement's positions. This is true, for example of anti-abortion protesters, who belong to a movement that targets health policy and practice. They often join the movement before they have clear views on abortion, attracted by social ties [13]. In turn, a movement's positions typically shift as new people join. Slogans on signs give unreliable indications of what any movement stands for.

Fifth, a movement is not merely composed of individuals. Epstein explains that the early social movement concerned with HIV/AIDS was "built on the foundation of the gay and lesbian movement" and its "pre-existing organizations." Once a health crisis struck the gay community, these organizations reconfigured themselves and developed a new agenda, including pressuring the FDA to approve drugs faster and with different criteria [5].

Some of today's movements profess a strong aversion to organizations and formal structures, presenting themselves as loose, voluntary networks of equals [14]. But even an extreme case of an anti-hierarchical movement, such as Occupy Wall Street, still develops procedures and structures that go beyond individuals.

Finally, movements do much more than protest. In fact, many seasoned grassroots leaders know that protests are mainly opportunities for recruiting people to do the more important work of a movement [15]. By organizing a march or a picket line, organizers attract allies, but then they take down names and contact information so they can call on people for other tasks. In addition to protesting, social movements organize strikes, occupations, and boycotts, raise money for litigation and ballot initiatives, recruit and support candidates for public office and leaders of private organizations, found new entities (including companies), produce knowledge, and educate.

How Institutions and Professionals Should View Movements

A more complex model of social movements should encourage people who hold positions inside institutions—including medical researchers, clinicians, and health administrators—to react to movements more analytically and more constructively.

It is not enough to assess a movement's current slogans or explicit demands, because the movement almost always harbors disagreements and is likely to shift. Nor is it enough to identify and consider engaging individuals who are associated with the movement. Almost all movements incorporate organizations as well as people. Indeed, one's *own* organization may be partly involved in a movement, to the extent that one's colleagues identify in various ways with it.

In order to decide whether and how to engage with a movement, a scientist or health professional must understand it. The main question is not whether the movement's slogans are congruent with current scientific consensus. It is also important to understand the movement's capacity for learning and growth.

I have been advocating the SPUD framework for assessing movements [16, 17]. In this framework, "S" stands for *scale*: movements should strive to recruit large numbers of individuals and groups, because they have more power if they are large. "P" stands for *pluralism*: movements are more effective and learn and react better if they encompass people with diverse perspectives, backgrounds, and social roles. "U" stands for *unity*: movements must come together behind shared demands at any given time, or else they can't make effective demands. And "D" stands for *depth*: movements must help their participants to grow in knowledge, skill, experience, and wisdom.

Unfortunately, scale and unity are in tension, because it is difficult to have both many members and deep learning experiences for all. And unity and pluralism conflict because it is hard to achieve a common position if a movement encompasses a wide diversity of backgrounds and perspectives. Figure 8.1 demonstrates these tradeoffs and can be used to assess the strengths and weaknesses of a movement at a given moment, understanding that all movements evolve over time.

I developed SPUD as a diagnostic tool for movements to use on themselves, but scientists and health professionals might consider similar criteria when they assess the movements that are targeting their issues and institutions.

If a movement is *unified,* then scientists may have to decide whether it is unified behind a platform that is congruent with scientific findings and a compelling theory of social justice. For example, if the movement labeled as the "anti-vaxxers" is truly defined by a common opposition to (all) vaccinations, then many scientists will feel compelled to resist it. But if a movement is not actually unified, then a scientific institution might subtly intervene by organizing forums on the movement's issues that incorporate multiple perspectives. No worthy movement will be threatened by an open debate.

On the other hand, if a movement is already *pluralist*, the institution should recognize that plurality. Broadly-engaged team scientists should demonstrate that they understand the range of views within the movement and the richness of its internal debate. They should avoid stereotyping movement participants.

If a movement is already providing *depth*, in the form of training programs, retreats, seminars, and reading groups, then scientific and health institutions might

Fig. 8.1 The SPUD Framework for Assessing Movements

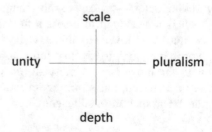

consider supporting and recognizing that learning. They could supply research findings and summaries for use in these programs and even consider awarding academic credentials for successful participation.

On the other hand, if a movement has achieved *scale*—recruiting many followers—but it does not offer *depth*, then a scientific institution can compensate by providing learning opportunities to complement the movement. Scientific organizations and disciplines can generate writing, research, and other academic work helps movement participants learn.

Scientific and health institutions have limited resources and face heavy demands. Therefore, it is important not to place unreasonable burdens on them to engage with social movements, particularly as movements proliferate. I do not think there exists a satisfactory body of practical tools and tips, although I offer SPUD as one contribution. It might make sense for scientists to identify participants in social movements who already have some scientific background and engage them first. But that is just a proposal; on the whole, the study of how scientists should engage with social movements is in its infancy.

Building Better Relationships Between Science and Social Movements

Laboratories, hospitals, universities, and scientific disciplines are not movements; they are institutions. Institutions can expect to be targeted by movements, which creates tension [9]. The question is often not whether to choose to form a "bidirectional relationship" with a stakeholder but how to deal with a movement at one's door.

Scientists and health professionals are accountable to professional bodies, state agencies, or trustees, not to movements. They must keep some distance from the movements that recruit their own patients, students, and employees. Also, when acting as educators, scientists should often strive for impartiality about the contested issues in our society and not use their classrooms to advocate or oppose any particular movements.

Notwithstanding these legitimate reasons to maintain some distance between science and social movements, there is much room for productive interchange. Building better relationships between science and social movements is especially important for broadly engaged team science, given its commitment to engagement. But engaging members of a movement is not just a question of reaching out to individuals as stakeholders. It requires a nuanced understanding of social movement dynamics and better practices for engaging movements productively.

References

1. Concannon TW, Meissner P, Grunbaum JA, McElwee N, Guise JM, Santa J, Conway PH, Daudelin D, Morrato EH, Leslie LK (2012) A new taxonomy for stakeholder engagement in patient-centered outcomes research. J Gen Intern Med 27(8):985–991. https://doi.org/10.1007/s11606-012-2037-1
2. Concannon TW, Grant S, Welch V, Petkovic J, Selby J, Crowe S, Synnot A, Greer-Smith R, Mayo-Wilson E, Tambor E, Tugwell P, Multi Stakeholder Engagement C (2019) Practical guidance for involving stakeholders in Health Research. J Gen Intern Med 34(3):458–463. https://doi.org/10.1007/s11606-018-4738-6
3. Patient-Centered Outcomes Research Institute (2021) https://www.pcori.org/engagement/engagement-resources. Accessed 8 Feb 2021
4. Arnstein S (1969) A ladder of citizen participation. J Am Inst Plann 35(4):216–224. https://doi.org/10.1080/01944366908977225
5. Epstein S (1995) The construction of lay expertise: AIDS activism and the forging of credibility in the reform of clinical trials. Sci Technol Human Values 20(4):408–437. https://doi.org/10.1177/016224399502000402
6. Allsop J, Jones K, Baggott R (2004) Health consumer groups in the UK: a new social movement? Sociol Health Illn 26(6):737–756. https://doi.org/10.1111/j.0141-9889.2004.00416.x
7. Caruso D (2010) Autism in the U.S.: social movement and legal change. Am J Law Med 36(4):483–539. https://doi.org/10.1177/009885881003600401
8. Atwell M, Bridgeland J, Levine P (2017) Civic Deserts: America's Civic Health Challenge. https://www.ncoc.org/wp-content/uploads/2017/10/2017CHIUpdate-FINAL-small.pdf
9. Caren N, Ghoshal RA, Ribas V (2011) A social movement generation: cohort and period trends in protest attendance and petition signing. Am Sociol Rev 76(1):125–151. https://doi.org/10.2307/25782183
10. McCarthy JD, Zald MN (1977) Resource mobilization and social movements: a partial theory. Am J Sociol 82(6):1212–1241
11. Aarons GA, Wells RS, Zagursky K, Fettes DL, Palinkas LA (2009) Implementing evidence-based practice in community mental health agencies: a multiple stakeholder analysis. Am J Public Health 99(11):2087–2095. https://doi.org/10.2105/AJPH.2009.161711
12. Tilly C (2004) Social movements, 1768–2004 / Charles Tilly. vol Accessed from https://nla.gov.au/nla.cat-vn3078808. Paradigm Publishers, Boulder, Col
13. Munson ZW (2008) The making of pro-life activists : how social movement mobilization works. University of Chicago Press, Chicago, Chicago
14. Bennett WL (2013) The logic of connective action : digital media and the personalization of contentious politics. Cambridge studies in contentious politics. Cambridge University Press, Cambridge. 40022730480
15. Hersh E (2020) Politics is for power : how to move beyond political hobbyism, take action, and make real change. Scribner, an imprint of Simon & Schuster, Inc, New York, NY
16. Levine P (2018) Habermas with a whiff of tear gas: nonviolent campaigns and deliberation in an era of authoritarianism. J Pub Deliberat 14(2)
17. Levine P (2019) The role of social movements in fostering sounder public judgement. Sounder Public Judgement Working Paper Series

Chapter 9
A Basic Scientist's Journey: Engaging Stakeholders Through Civic Science

Jonathan A. Garlick

Abstract Civic Science offers an actionable framework that helps scientists work collectively with citizens through a participatory process that reaches out to community members and other stakeholders as authentic and integral partners of their broadly engaged research teams. As a new approach that reaches beyond traditional disciplinary boundaries, Civic Science can support collaborative partnerships across the scientific community and with individuals and groups from different contexts. In this chapter, I will discuss how Civic Science provided me with an action- and skill-based framework that supported my transition to greater engagement of stakeholders in my research. It offered a way to connect the potential benefits of my research discoveries with a wide spectrum of stakeholders, and it provided new skills, partnerships, attitudes, and processes that supported me in this broad civic engagement with science and communities that science serves. I learned that Civic Science could connect a more inclusive, collectivist basic science lab with many communities and citizens, including the patients I hoped my research would benefit. Essentially, Civic Science had a dramatic impact on my research and changed me by helping me apply principles and practice for achieving science for the public good. It changed me from a basic scientist in my lab to a basic scientist in society by cineections my research discoveries to the communities and patients they are meant to serve.

Keywords Civic science · Broadly engaged team science · Scleroderma patients · Stakeholders

Civic science is a set of framework and practices that can help scientists working in any discipline become more outward facing [1]. The work of basic scientists—those working in the earliest stages of clinical discovery—can benefit from the practice of

J. A. Garlick (✉)
Tufts Initiative in Civic Science at Tufts University School of Dental Medicine, Boston, MA, USA

Tufts Clinical and Translational Science Institute, Boston, MA, USA
e-mail: jonathan.garlick@tufts.edu

© The Author(s), under exclusive license to Springer Nature Switzerland AG 2022
D. Lerner et al. (eds.), *Broadly Engaged Team Science in Clinical and Translational Research*, https://doi.org/10.1007/978-3-030-83028-1_9

Civic Science in concrete ways. My own story illustrates how the practice of Civic Science can have a dramatic impact on basic science discovery.

Civic Science reaches out across disciplinary boundaries engaging scientists representing diverse types of knowledge and expertise as well as to community members, policy makers, and patients engaging them as authentic and integral partners on their teams. Through Civic Science, scientists become more "community literate" while learning what individuals and communities think and feel about scientific ideas. It does this by offering an actionable framework that helps scientists work collectively with non-scientists [1].

A central goal of Civic Science is to bridge the persistent gap between actions taken to generate scientific knowledge and those involved in translating that knowledge into improved human health and well-being. Rather than viewing communication with the public as a one-way dissemination of scientific information, Civic Science advocates for approaches to communication that build relationships of dialogue and trust with citizens. These partnerships grow when scientists learn to facilitate an exchange of information with individuals who differ from themselves in their values, beliefs, and power and to respect the knowledge, experience, and identities of citizens and communities with and without scientific credentials. Civic Science entails a commitment to building and sustaining productive, bi-directional relationships between scientists and the citizens they hope to serve throughout the research process.

Civic Science draws from research and theory in diverse fields such as science communication, civic advocacy, social action, civic organization, civic dialogue, deliberative practices, science and technology studies (STS), and civic studies [1–3]. The goals of Civic Science evolved as a response to the need to pursue scientific knowledge that better aligns with societal interests, both to increase citizens' trust in science and make science a more collaborative undertaking [4]. The field of Civic Science offers a blueprint for new kinds of collaborations where citizens can enhance scientific inquiry by integrating local, indigenous knowledge [1, 5–7].

In this chapter, I will discuss how Civic Science provided me with an action- and skill-based framework that supported greater engagement of stakeholders in my research. In this journey with Civic Science, I was able to instill a more inclusive, collectivist culture in my basic science lab that would bring greater value to many communities and citizens, including the patients I hoped my research would benefit. Ultimately, Civic Science had a dramatic impact on my research and changed me from a basic scientist in my lab to a basic scientist in society.

Learning that External Stakeholders Are Essential to a Basic Scientist

My journey with Civic Science began 10 years ago with a breakthrough moment that propelled me into understanding that I could no longer work alone in the silo of my lab. As a stem cell researcher studying diabetic wound healing, I work with cells sampled from patients (patient-derived cells). But on August 23, 2010, a court ruling froze all federal funding for human embryonic stem cell research, including mine.

I was completely blindsided by this legal ruling, as I was unaware of the simmering political, ethical, and legal controversies surrounding the use of human embryos for stem cell research. While I puzzled through the question of what would happen to my research as a result of this ruling, I realized that I had not considered how my basic research was directly connected to the lives of many stakeholders that were part of the decision to freeze federal funding. It was a wake-up call to begin understanding how I might address some of the roadblocks that were limiting the impact of my translational research.

This initial breakthrough moment was underscored a short time later when once again my basic science research seemed too siloed and socially isolated. I felt that I had good ideas, but I was missing a truly integrated, collaborative team with whom I could brainstorm and execute research with a more palpable translational impact. Unfortunately, my grant proposal reviewers often agreed, and my track record for funding needed to improve. I had to figure out how to leverage the strengths and expertise of researchers trained in different, but related fields and to bridge the disciplinary cultures that define them. I also needed to invite in new stakeholders to build more holistic research teams—including patient communities, drug discovery experts, and/or start-up ventures—through which my basic research projects could become more applied and translational. I longed to create team-based collaborations that could lead to the development of new treatments and interventions to improve the lives patients suffering from the rare diseases we studied.

Another breakthrough moment came over a lunchtime conversation with Dr. Michael Whitfield, a very talented genomics researcher at Dartmouth School of Medicine, while we were at a Scleroderma Patient Education Conference. It quickly became clear that we would be great collaborators because he could do something I couldn't do (genomics), and I could do something he couldn't do (tissue engineering human skin). At the same time, I was inspired by the scleroderma patients I met at this conference. They came to learn new information about treatments, research, and living with scleroderma, and after several conversations with these individuals, I needed to look no further for patients who could donate cells to my basic research studies. By the time I left the conference, 20 patients had signed up to give their blood and skin for my research. That alone was a critically important advance for a basic scientist studying a rare disease. However, what started as a group of patients who were participants in our research studies changed to collaborators and research team members in broadly engaged team science.

Growing our Broadly Engaged Team Science Approach

In the weeks following the scleroderma conference, we rapidly grew a team-based research group aimed at translating my basic, early-stage innovations by moving them toward the drug discovery market. My research team visited scleroderma patients at their Scleroderma Support Groups in Massachusetts and New Hampshire and word quickly spread among them that our research needed their partnership.

Our plan was to engineer miniature skin-like tissues with scleroderma patients' cells to create a drug screening tool that could be used to discover new drugs to treat scleroderma and fibrosis. Our research team soon included patients and their families who had signed up to donate their cells. In addition, our group included Dartmouth collaborators, clinical researchers, and an early-stage biotech start-up that was planning to develop and market the engineered skin we created—all of whom I met and networked with at scleroderma patient education meetings. Over the last three years, our team has received one million in Small Business Research Grants from the National Institutes of Health (NIH) to engineer skin that can be widely used as a patient skin-like platform to screen potential drugs to treat scleroderma. I believe that securing these translational grants was strongly supported by engaging networks of scleroderma patients, which provided important evidence that "end-users" needed and wanted the results of our discoveries.

A broadly engaged team science approach enabled me to address multiple stages of stakeholder engagement, often in unexpected ways. For instance, I was able to network and brainstorm about the scope of the study with our patient community, which informed an understanding of strategies for patient recruitment through their network of patient support groups. In addition, strategizing with leadership of our Small Business Innovation Research (SBIR) partner was critical to idea generation about how our engineered skins could be commercialized and disseminated, and our Dartmouth partners were able to offer crucial insights into the reproducibility of our tissue fabrication process by offering whole genome analyses of all tissues generated.

With this newly acquired awareness, I was able to use a variety of methods to ensure that all stakeholder voices were valued and to continually clarify the benefits and impact of open communication to all community members and researchers on our team. First, by networking with this patient community and participating alongside them and their families in "Walks for Scleroderma," we embedded a culture of care and collaboration into our team science approach. My graduate students drew inspiration from getting to know who was donating the cells they were studying in the lab. Secondly, individuals with scleroderma donated skin and blood and then came to our lab to see, for the first time, how research is conducted. During one of these visits, a patient said to us, "I understand now how this works. We give you cells, you give us hope." It was incredibly motivating to everyone in my lab to hear this.

Learning the Importance of Adopting New Communication Practices

Successfully engaging patients and their families in my basic research studies involved overcoming several barriers. First, I did not know if the scleroderma patient community would be interested in engaging with a scientist whose discoveries might seem distant to their immediate needs for care and support. Secondly, I thought that the time needed to connect with this patient community would put pressure on graduate students and staff who already were busy with their projects. Finally, I was not certain that the funding agencies would value expanding our research team to include patients at the earliest stages of our basic science research project. Over time, all of these concerns proved unfounded. I also learned that these are frequently assumed barriers and not significant challenges that could not be overcome.

I was highly motivated to ensure that my basic science discoveries would help patients. So, I relied on my scleroderma patient collaborators to teach me how my results could impact their health and well-being. After all, who understood what it meant to live with scleroderma better than they did? Through informal conversations, I learned what scleroderma patients found most challenging in their daily lives and what gave them hope. These patients contributed to our research team through the strong personal connections that developed between them and my grad students and staff. They were a key component in building the atmosphere of understanding needed for us to share our passions, our common vision, and our love for what we were doing.

I also found that building effective communication with diverse stakeholders through our team-based collaborations was a two-way street. My basic research was addressing fundamental questions using sophisticated tissue engineering approaches, genomic tools, and epigenetic analyses that were not always understandable to researchers in other disciplines. To build greater stakeholder engagement, I needed to communicate the impact of my research to my collaborators, and they needed to communicate with me how they might apply these findings in their own disciplines. For example, it was critical to our clinical collaborators that we establish that the clinical subtypes seen in scleroderma patients would need to be reproduced in our skin tissue models of scleroderma. As a result, I shifted our tissue fabrication approach to sample patient skin biopsies from a much broader range of patients than I had originally planned. I learned that cross-disciplinary communication was a critical aspect of successful broadly engaged team science.

I was able to overcome some of the communication challenges I faced by striking a balance between different forms of knowledge, information, and preferences held by different stakeholders. I realized the need for effective communication that supported hearing all team members to develop a shared vision with them, and I learned to understand the challenges that our clinical collaborators faced when working with a patient population that had incredibly complex and diverse clinical presentations resulting from the multiple organ systems that were affected by scleroderma. I worked closely to learn the challenges that our biotech start-up partner faced when thinking about how to scale up our lab-made skin. Perhaps, most importantly, I learned that the scleroderma patient community was an ideal community with whom to build this shared vision. They were very active in organizing educational symposia and patient support groups, and they were eager to invite my lab and my collaborators to learn about the needs of the scleroderma community together with them.

In some ways, I feel that I have rebranded my role as a basic scientist by carefully mapping out opportunities for collaboration with previously unimagined stakeholders. I transitioned to a new research approach that led to a redirection, reformulation, and restating of my research objective. I did this by planning experiments that had the needs of the scleroderma patient community as our goal, and by creating skin-like tissues that closely mimicked individual patients. This shift to a different vision of a more personalized approach to patient care has accelerated the translation of my basic research in ways that have supported its potential health impacts. I had been trying for many years to find ways to make my 3D tissue engineered models of human skin available to the drug development community. Although the lab-made skin we engineered had been adopted by many basic scientists, finding a niche where I could direct these tissues to broader utilization or even commercialization to the drug discovery community had remained elusive.

By reimagining my identity as a basic researcher, I was able to more effectively identify and communicate with teams of diverse stakeholders regarding complex scientific projects. I have learned that it is possible for other basic scientists to find ways to share their expertise with a broad range of stakeholders to improve their readiness to collaborate in ways that capture the wisdom of all partners. To basic scientists, it is possible to build highly interactive and integrated research teams that will translate their basic discoveries to improve the health of patients they hope to serve. This can be done by reaching out to diverse groups of stakeholders and using effective communication strategies to build more inclusive research teams. Beyond this, another beneficial outcome is that this can become a springboard to address concerns about patient participation in clinical trials. This will also increase the likelihood that investigators will have an impact on patients through their increased participation in clinical research trials, increased health care access, and more optimal drug safety and efficacy testing. Most importantly, early-stage investigators can develop communication skills that can build trust and transparency with a range of stakeholders to address community concerns relevant to the translation of their basic science discoveries.

A Path Forward out of the Silos: A Civic Science Framework that Supports Broadly Engaged Team Science

Civic Science offered me a framework to overcome the reservations and fears I faced about reaching across boundaries to develop relationships between my lab and the people I hoped to serve with my research. I was able to learn and apply a participatory approach to research that respected the knowledge, experience, and identities of people and communities without scientific credentials. Through my trainings in science communication at Tufts and with the dialogue group Essential Partners [8], I was able to develop skills that helped me engage and communicate more effectively with other scientists and community-based stakeholders as my research became more outward facing.

Essentially, Civic Science seeks to shift the training, practice, and experience of scientists by providing new insights and skills that help them reimagine their professional identity through a civic lens. First, it helps scientists to better understand the benefits of engaging individuals without scientific credentials to build shared understandings and solutions on scientific issues. For example, I learned to hold my "expertise lightly" and to hone my listening skills; to appreciate different forms of knowledge and preferences held by diverse stakeholders. Second, it orients scientists and their institutions to the importance of committing to equity and inclusion at all levels of the scientific enterprise. These commitments are important to safeguarding against the marginalization of citizens and to ensure that science is representative of the people it intends to serve. Third, Civic Science embraces bi-directional communication approaches that build relationships of dialogue and trust with individuals and institutions. These partnerships grow when scientists learn to facilitate an exchange of information among individuals that differ in their values, beliefs, and power. Fourth, it promotes skills needed to build relationships that support an outward-facing research approach. These skills have helped me to feel more confident to build networks of practice with citizens, patients, and other stakeholders through collaborative engagement. I have found new ways to communicate more effectively across barriers that had limited effective stakeholder engagement and productive interdisciplinary collaborations in the past. Finally, Civic Science skills help scientists to mobilize and engage others in research. Research sponsors are increasingly interested in scientists who can effectively reach across boundaries to engage stakeholders as authentic and integral members of my research team.

I relied on Civic Science to support developing my skills in creating an inclusive environment in my basic research agenda. These skills are starting to be incoproated into university cirricula, classrooms, and scientific training so that early-stage researchers can learn that relationship-building, listening, and considering a diverse array of nuanced narratives is an essential part of the scientific process and not an afterthought [9]. It has become clear to me that basic scientists tranined with Civic Science skills will be more adept at building research teams as authentic partners in their research.

Disruptions in my research due to a federal court ruling and a lack of funding on my collaborative grants caused me to take a step back and think more broadly. This happened at the same time as I was encountering opportunities for Civic Science training. These forces worked together to bring me to a place of a more broadly engaged, team approach to science. While I understood that science appropriately rewards and values individualistic efforts which are essential for scientific breakthroughs, I now understand that such individualism has limitations for addressing complex, interdisciplinary research questions that have meaningful human dimensions. Civic Science offers scientists skills to shift the culture of their science to a more collectivistic mindset. Over time I began to understand that the acquisition of science communication and outreach skills at critical stages of one's career development can impact the inclusivity of our basic research in ways that can shift the culture of science to a more holistic practice.

Now, I routinely work to engage stakeholders in the broadest sense through my basic research. I learned that stakeholder engagement emerges through the bi-directional communication between members of my basic science research team and these stakeholders, and I continually seek new ways to include individuals or groups that would be directly impacted by my basic science discoveries. Many of the scientific issues that arose early in my career were linked to systemic barriers related to marginalization and bias on the basis of gender identity and expression, socioeconomic status, race, and other identities. I trained to communicate in ways that could build bridges by learning dialogue skills to better facilitate discourse on science issues through the lens of identity and the dynamics of power and privilege. I found that I could achieve a path forward by aligning my lab's research goals with this more inclusive communication approach that could build trust and transparency with potential research partners at the outset of our research, rather than having challenges arise later on.

Reaching out to new stakeholders had a large impact on my decision-making about the conduct and direction of our basic research program. As a result, I have been able to benefit from building holistic research teams that have included diverse stakeholders and community members from the outset of our work as authentic and active partners in our research. This has included working with patient support groups, their families and communities, drug developers, start-up companies and policy makers. As a result, my stem cell research lab has taken on new and unex-pected dimensions by building research teams with diverse skills and different types of knowledge. My lab became better positioned for translation, by having access to a large spectrum of patient cells that we could test in our tissue engineered skin as a drug screening platform. These skills helped me to more effectively connect with teams of diverse stakeholders on T0 (basic research) and T.5 (pre-clinical testing before translation to human) stages of my research. The rationale for involvement in each of these stages was based on the need to share expertise with a broad range of stakeholders to improve the readiness for everyone to collaborate in ways that will capture the wisdom of all partners. Our work also gained increased clinical rele-vance through our communication with patient communities. This enabled my research lab to more fully realize our longer-range, translational research goal of delivering drugs to patients while supporting more immediate goals such as procur-ing much-needed patient-derived cells and funding from sources that appreciated the inclusion of patients in our basic science research.

Looking Towards the Future of Civic Science as a Transformational Force in Science

There is an urgent need to capture the imagination of early-stage scientists-in-training about the importance of defining their professional activities through a more holistic lens. A culture of Civic Science educates and trains scientists through-out their career development with formative civic skills that offer foundations for their career decisions and actions. This includes that can build inclusive research teams that can become springboards to address community concerns about patient participation in clinical research trials, increase health care access and affordability, concerns and provide the public witrh accessible information about the translation of basic discovery, to better understand how this benefits their health [1].

But how can we make the case in our university departments and schools that our basic science processes and outcomes can be viewed as a force for societal impact and change? Civic Science helps to create connections across boundaries that are often reinforced by prevailing structures within our institutions.

To more fully cultivate initiatives that value citizen knowledge, our institutions may need to change work incentives and structures. Innovative teaching and research approaches may be needed for institutions to offer resources for scientists to connect to the civic dimensions of their research programs. This may require rebranding the role of the scientist as an "outward-facing" citizen, whose "broadly-engaged" work will result in higher quality teaching, research and learning that can prepare them to lead lives of responsible citizenship linked to meaningful personal and professional development. Through my own experience, I have learned that basic research that crosses disciplinary and community boundaries can lead to new transdisciplinary and interdisciplinary funding streams. Building funding streams based on broadly engaged basic research will make the case to institutional leadership that creating alternative, actionable, and inclusive systems will help guide changes in incentives and rules that currently guide the way science is done.

For junior investigators who are not in control of their own labs to adopt these lessons they must first become aware of the channels of communication that can open doors and help flatten destructive power differentials that exist within institutions. A second step is to leverage these channels of communication to make the case that a vibrant culture of broadly engaged science can build momentum in institutions in ways that will win the support of federal funding agencies and other organizations that already understand the multifaceted institutional role of science in this broader context. By creating programs and partnerships within and across our institutions, Civic Science is opening new opportunities for changes in institutional incentives and processes that can best support basic science research programs and train and prepare scientists to productively and broadly engage with their community- or patient-based partners.

Civic Science informs skill sets that are not traditionally incorporated into scientific training. However, performing outward-facing, basic research should not fall on the shoulders of a small group of scientists who do the heavy lifting because their personal experiences have given them a stake in engaging more directly with citizens and stakeholders. Rather, scientific institutions need to generalize this work as trainees proceed in their careers. In this light, the need for embedding stakeholder engagement is pressing. If basic scientists at an early stage in their career perceive that institutional values do not align with their own, they may exit their careers before they fully realize the promise of the incredibly rewarding careers that have an outward-facing dimension.

References

1. Garlick JA, Levine P (2017) Where civics meets science: building science for the public good through civic science. Oral Dis 23(6):692–696. https://doi.org/10.1111/odi.12534
2. Spencer JP (2015) Reflections of a civic scientist. In: Boyte HC (ed) Democracy's education. public work, citizenship, and the future of colleges and universities. Vanderbilt University Press, pp 211–220. https://doi.org/10.2307/j.ctv1675bg2.26
3. Christopherson EG, Dietram AS, Brooke S (2018) The civic science imperative. Stanford Social Innovat Rev 16(2):46–52
4. Sarewitz D (2017) Science and the cultivation of public judgment. Connect Ann J Kettering Foundat:67–71
5. Wynne B (1992) Misunderstood misunderstanding: social identities and public uptake of science. Pub Understand Sci (Bristol, England) 1(3):281–304. https://doi.org/10.1088/0963-6625/1/3/004
6. Epstein S (1995) The construction of lay expertise: aids activism and the forging of credibility in the reform of clinical trials. Sci Technol Human Values 20(4):408–437. https://doi.org/10.1177/016224399502000402
7. Fortun K, Fortun M (2005) Scientific imaginaries and ethical plateaus in contemporary U.S. toxicology. Am Anthropol 107(1):43–54. https://doi.org/10.1525/aa.2005.107.1.043
8. Sarrouf J, Hyten K (2019) Creating cultures of dialogue in higher education: stories and lessons from essential partners. In: Longo NV, Shaffer TJ (ed) Creating space for democracy: a primer on dialogue and deliberation in higher education
9. Garlick, J (2021) The pandemic, Trustworthiness and a place for Civic Science in higher education. in Higher Education Exchange. The Kettering Foundation. In press

Chapter 10
Lessons in Public Involvement from Across the Pond

Marisha E. Palm, Tina Coldham, and David Evans

Abstract Broadly engaged team science has the potential to change how health care research is conducted. It encourages a more inclusive approach, with an expanded base of knowledge and expertise consulted. However, successfully engaging a broader study team to conduct research requires thoughtful guidance and supportive infrastructure. This chapter briefly outlines the development and evolution of public involvement in health research in England and compares and contrasts this with the progression of public involvement in the US. England has been at the forefront of the movement towards more inclusive health research teams, and in the last decade the US has increasingly invested in infrastructure to encourage and support public involvement. We consider the lessons from England and the US and discuss how broadly engaged team science could complement and build on the efforts to support public involvement in health research.

Keywords Health care systems · Health care research · Public involvement · Stakeholder engagement

Broadly engaged team science has the potential to change how health care research is conducted. It encourages a more inclusive approach, with an expanded base of knowledge and expertise consulted. However, successfully engaging a broader study team to conduct research requires thoughtful guidance and supportive infrastructure. This chapter briefly outlines the development and evolution of public

M. E. Palm (✉)
Institute for Clinical Research and Health Policy Studies, Tufts Medical Center, Boston, MA, USA

Tufts Clinical and Translational Research Institute, Boston, MA, USA
e-mail: mpalm@tuftsmedicalcenter.org

T. Coldham
Participation, Involvement, and Engagement Advisor to NIHR CED, England, UK

D. Evans
University of the West of England, Bristol, UK

© The Author(s), under exclusive license to Springer Nature Switzerland AG 2022
D. Lerner et al. (eds.), *Broadly Engaged Team Science in Clinical and Translational Research*, https://doi.org/10.1007/978-3-030-83028-1_10

involvement in health research in England and compares and contrasts this with the progression of public involvement in the US. England has been at the forefront of the movement towards more inclusive health research teams, and in the last decade the US has increasingly invested in infrastructure to encourage and support public involvement. We consider the lessons from England and the US and discuss how broadly engaged team science could complement and build on the efforts to support public involvement in health research.

INVOLVE Definitions:

Public:

- The term public includes patients, potential patients, care[give]rs, and people who use health and social care services, as well as people from organizations that represent people who use services.

Involvement:

- Research being carried out "with" or "by" members of the public rather than "to," "about," or "for" them.

Public Involvement in Health Research in England

The importance of public involvement in health research was first acknowledged in the 1991 English National Healthcare System (NHS) Research and Development Strategy [1]. Five years later, in 1996, the English Department of Health established Consumers in NHS Research (renamed INVOLVE in 2003), which went on to serve as the national hub for public involvement in health research. INVOLVE became part of the National Institute for Health Research (NIHR), the nation's largest funder of health, public health, and social care research, from its establishment in 2006 until April 2020, when it was incorporated into the new NIHR Centre for Engagement and Dissemination. Since the inclusion of public involvement in health research within NHS policy, followed by the establishment of a hub to promote this work, public involvement in research has grown significantly [2]. This support for involvement has been cemented in further policy documents; in 2001, involvement across health care and research became a statutory requirement in the England under the Health and Social Care Act, and in 2006 Department of Health guidance made clear that "patients and the public must be involved in all stages of the research process" [3].

The NIHR was established to improve the health and wealth of England through research, and it is now one of the most integrated health research systems in the world [4]. The NIHR works in partnership with the NHS, universities, local governments, and other research funders, as well as patients and the public, to provide support and resources for health research and scientific advancement. In addition to the key role that INVOLVE has played in health research in England, there are a number of other parts of the NIHR that actively involve members of the public in their support and/or funding of health care research. These include but are not limited to:

- the NIHR Central Commissioning Facility (CCF), which manages five NIHR research programs, the Research Design Service, and several NIHR infrastructure schemes [5];
- the James Lind Alliance (JLA) Priority Setting Partnerships (PSPs), which bring public members (patients, care[give]rs) and clinicians together to identify and prioritize treatment uncertainties [5];
- the Health Technology Assessment (HTA) Program, which funds research about the impact of health care treatments and tests [6]; and
- the Research Design Service (RDS), which provides support to health and social care researchers who are writing grants [2, 7].

An assessment of progress in public involvement in NIHR research entitled the "Breaking Boundaries Review" began in 2014 and involved patients and the public, funders, and national and international partners [9]. An online survey, evidence sessions, workshop events, and existing systematic reviews were collected to assess progress and develop a vision looking toward 2025. An overview published in 2015 extolled the NIHR as a global leader in making public involvement a core principle and advanced a vision for the future that highlighted co-production of knowledge [10]. It also included a recommendation that co-production be explored in further detail and new guidance was recently published, including key principles and features. In this guidance, co-producing a research project is defined as "an approach in which researchers, practitioners, and the public work together, sharing power and responsibility from the start to the end of the project, including the generation of knowledge" [9].

In addition to NIHR support for public involvement, there are a number of non-NIHR bodies that support health research in England and involve the public. For example, the National Institute for Health and Care Excellence (NICE) aims to improve health outcomes by producing evidence-based guidance and developing quality standards and performance metrics for those providing and commissioning health and care services [14, 15]. The Health Research Authority (HRA) protects and promotes the interests of the public in health and social care research and seeks to ensure that research meets ethical standards [14]. Plus, several charities that support and fund health research also involve the public in their work (e.g., Cancer Research UK, British Heart Foundation, Wellcome Trust) [15–17]. Together, the NIHR and other organizations that support health research in England have partnered to embed public involvement at all stages of research. Public members play key decision-making roles in regulatory bodies, sitting on local ethics committees, engaging in development of NICE guidelines, and being part of grant funding review boards. The importance of including public members as part of health and social care research teams has also been emphasized; the majority of NIHR funding streams require public involvement, requesting involvement plans and budget information within the grant and details of involvement in the annual grant reporting.

Traditionally, NIHR INVOLVE defined *public involvement* as "research being carried out 'with' or 'by' members of the public rather than 'to,' 'about,' or 'for' them" [18]. This was seen as distinct from *public engagement*, where information about research is provided and disseminated to members of the public and communities, and from *participation*, where members of the public are recruited to take part as subjects in a research study. It is unclear whether the new NIHR Centre for Engagement and Dissemination (CED) will redefine the word *engagement* to mean active bidirectional communication as well as unidirectional provision of information. As communication evolves, the NIHR seeks to engage with more people digitally, interacting with the public on platforms such as Twitter and revisiting its Digital Strategy to bring it up to date [19]. There is precedent for using the term "engagement" to cover a wider range of activity; the Patient-Centered Outcomes Research Institute (PCORI) in the United States uses engagement to mean "the involvement of patients, caregivers, clinicians, insurers, and others across the healthcare community in every aspect of the research process" [19].

The Role and Evolution of INVOLVE

The structures and organizations around INVOLVE have changed in the nearly quarter century since its inception as Consumers in NHS Research, and they are now changing again. It is important to note that INVOLVE began and remained embedded within the primary health research funding body in the nation, recently becoming combined within a new center that still sits at the heart of the NIHR. This central positioning has enabled INVOLVE to influence decision-making around public involvement within the NIHR. INVOLVE has supported increased, inclusive public involvement across the range of NIHR activities, and its role as a centralized resource encouraging researchers to involve the public has helped England develop useful resources and guidelines in a co-produced and thoughtful manner since the early 2000s [20, 21]. This has given public involvement in health research a strong foundation in England and has heavily influenced other devolved nations' approaches to public involvement in health research. The new NIHR Centre was launched in 2020, and its website promises to build on the work of INVOLVE, with all of its activities underpinned by public involvement [23].

Since the NIHR CED was only recently launched, we focus here on the three main roles that INVOLVE has played to date. The first role was development and provision of guidance and resources to support involvement of the public in research, as defined above. This ranged from "how to" guidance, to standards of practice, reimbursement rates, and training for researchers as well as members of the public. The second role was advising the wider NIHR on public involvement, as funding streams were established and developed, and as guidance was created for the involvement of the public in the development of grants and the conduct of research. Experts within INVOLVE and its advisory group provided guidance, set standards, and ensured involvement in the larger research structures as well as more contained research programs and projects. The third role was individual advice provision, where researchers were able to seek involvement advice as they were completing a grant application or deciding how to navigate reimbursement of public members. INVOLVE has played pivotal roles that the CED is likely to take up in future; however, it is notable that while it has supported guidance and infrastructure around public involvement, it has not served to fund health research.

The governance structure of INVOLVE was comprised of an Advisory Group, Executive Group, and Associate members. The INVOLVE Advisory Group had between 13 and 17 stakeholder members including a chair, and the Group was a broad mix of public members and health professionals and researchers, with the intention to ensure that the Group was diverse and inclusive [24]. The Group was established to provide an independent perspective, advising the Director of INVOLVE, and it was empowered to challenge and advise on INVOLVE's strategic direction and work program. Recruitment to the Advisory Group was an open and public process, with a clear role description, an application requirement, and an interview panel including public members. Three members of the Advisory Group were represented in the smaller Executive Group alongside the Director, INVOLVE staff, and two to three Regional Design Service Directors. They focused on the organizational strategy and on particular activities, e.g., achieving greater diversity, accepting new and innovative approaches, and adopting new technologies for effective public involvement. Associate members were those individuals who had served their full terms on the Advisory Group, but who remained available as a wider pool of people to assist INVOLVE in particular projects according to their skill set. The new Centre has disbanded the standing Advisory Group, with a view to starting with a newly selected group that initially will prioritize seldom heard voices in the general population within research. Its full functions are yet to be articulated and have been understandably delayed by COVID prioritization.

Public Involvement Resources

Resources developed by INVOLVE have traditionally been co-produced by working groups formed as sub-sets of the larger Advisory Group. They have resulted in tools that are publicly available via the INVOLVE website and in paper form for those without computer or internet access. The INVOLVE library is one of the cornerstones of its work in that these resources are co-produced, developed according to issues of importance to the research and involvement communities, and made accessible to all. Public involvement is highly contextual and there is no single best or right way to involve people in research, therefore many of the resources provide several examples that show the range and diversity of involvement activities and allow people to consider many possibilities (Table 10.1). At the time of writing, these resources can still be found on the INVOLVE website (www.invo.org.uk); the new Center will be selecting and moving them to the NIHR website in time, so they will remain publicly available and accessible [25].

Table 10.1 Public involvement resources and brief descriptions

Resources	Description
Jargon buster	A searchable glossary of words and definitions for some of the terms often used in public involvement in research
Public information pack	A booklet for people who want to find out more about getting involved in NHS, public health, and social care research
How to involve people in research	Information for researchers, including what is public involvement, why involve members of the public, how to involve members of the public, how to find people, and what to do if things go wrong
Payment and recognition for involvement	An introduction to good practice, an overview of budgeting for involvement, examples of payment policies, and a link to a benefits regulations and advice service
Guidance on co-producing research	Guidance including key principles and features of co-producing a research project and challenges that will need to be addressed in order for researchers, practitioners and the public to share power and responsibility
Resource center with libraries of references	Public involvement evidence library, resources for people planning public involvement, library of research projects that include public involvement, INVOLVE publications, library of public involvement examples
Learning and development	Guidance on how to plan and develop training and support for research panel members, project advisory group members, project steering group members, public reviewers, and peer interviewers
UK standards for public involvement	A multi-stakeholder effort providing clear statements of effective public involvement to allow improvement to be assessed over time

Compare and Contrast with Public Involvement in the US

The US population is larger than England's by a factor of nearly six, there is no national health care delivery system, the health care research funding structures are broader, and the function to support public involvement in health care research is less centralized. The US National Institutes of Health (NIH), which acts as a research funder but not a provider of care, established a Director's Council of Public Representatives (COPR) in 1998 to support public accountability via two-way communication with the public, encouraging public input, and providing information from the NIH to the public. The COPR is a Federal Advisory Committee that is comprised of 21 members of the public, defined broadly as: patients and family members of patients; health professionals; members of patient advocacy groups; those who work or volunteer in health care; communicators in health care; scientists; and academics [26]. Twelve years after COPR was formed, in 2010, the Patient-Centered Outcomes Research Institute (PCORI) was established as part of the US Patient Protection and Affordable Care Act [22, 27, 28]. PCORI funds patient-centered comparative clinical effectiveness research. It has also made strides in the 10 years since it was established to develop frameworks and advance the science and practice of patient-centered outcomes research. It performs a variety of different functions, including: funding a portfolio of research; holding an annual meeting; providing training and resources; maintaining a tool for published articles; facilitating local, regional, and national forums; recruiting and training public reviewers; and hosting a peer-to-peer repository of articles [29]. In addition to the work that PCORI does to support public involvement, the NIH and its foundations also promote public outreach and conduct special programs to involve the public in health research.

One difference between INVOLVE and PCORI is that PCORI has a more pro-scribed focus on comparative clinical effectiveness research, while INVOLVE has had a wider remit that encompasses all of health care research, as well as research into social care and public health beginning in 2001. INVOLVE was established to support active public involvement in research and was part of an integrated and comprehensive national health care system that has evolved to embed public involvement into many of its core health research structures and organizations. PCORI was established to fund patient-centered comparative clinical effectiveness research, with a mission to promote research guided by patients, caregivers, and the broader community. PCORI hosts PCORnet, an integrated partnership representing a diverse group of patients and organizations that serves to advance patient-centered research, engaging patients and caregivers as coequal collaborators with health pro-fessionals. It also makes investments in research infrastructure (e.g., Eugene Washington Engagement Awards), and acts as a national model and public involve-ment catalyst for other health care research bodies such as the US Food and Drug Administration (FDA) and the Centers for Medicare & Medicaid Services (CMS), as well as smaller research groups within universities [29].

The governance of INVOLVE and PCORI have both been intentionally inclu-sive, but in different ways. The governance of INVOLVE has been handled by "a broad mix of individuals who use health and social care services, care[give]rs, peo-ple from voluntary organizations, and health service and social care practitioners, managers, and researchers" [30]. The governance of PCORI is diversified across stakeholder groups, including patients, physicians and providers, private payers, employer purchasers, pharmaceutical, device, and diagnostic manufacturers or developers, quality improvement or health services researchers, and the federal gov-ernment [28]. These differences reflect the differences in health care systems and approaches to public health between the two countries.

The development and provision of public involvement materials has also been approached differently. Traditionally, the INVOLVE Executive Group and Advisory Group have worked to prioritize topical issues on which to focus and develop guid-ance and resources. INVOLVE resources were co-produced by sub-groups of the wider Advisory Group, consisting of researchers, practitioners, and the public. In addition, accessibility is emphasized, ensuring paper copies of materials for those who did not have computers, and plain English versions of the text in order to maxi-mize the number of people able to understand the guidance. PCORI has an Advisory Panel approved by their Board of Governors that provides expertise and offers input to ensure high standards and patient-centeredness [29]. PCORI's Engagement Rubric was developed collaboratively with their Advisory Panel. It is less apparent how their Advisory Panel or other members of the public are involved in the development of other engagement resources focused on training and reimbursement, suggesting that this may vary between resources or be decided on a case-by-case basis.

It is notable that, despite the differences between the research structures and the history of stakeholder involvement in the US and England, much of the guidance that has been developed is focused on similar topics, and many of the challenges that come with involvement work are the same on both slides of the Atlantic. Issues around recognition of public partners and figuring out systems for reimbursement (see PCORI's compensation framework [31] and INVOLVE's payment and recognition for public involvement [25]), distinguishing between participation and active involvement (see INVOLVE's jargon buster [25] and PCORI's glossary and engagement rubric [20, 32]), and training or facilitating researchers and members of the public to work together (see INVOLVE's developing training and support guidance [25] and PCORI's Research Fundamentals Training [29]) are very similar. The fact that these issues are difficult in multiple settings across very different health care and health research systems suggests that public involvement faces the same challenges in both countries. Acknowledging these similarities and the importance of countries learning from one another, the International Network for Public Involvement and Engagement in Health and Social Care Research was launched in London in 2017 and included INVOLVE and PCORI as well as similar organizations from other countries. Work has begun to establish a broad partnership that will share learnings and support public involvement globally, focused as a priority on training, standards and policies, guidelines, and impact [33].

What Can the US Learn from England?

England established systems that require rather than request the inclusion of the public voice in health care systems and health care research [34, 35]. These requirements have been followed by the development of resources that help researchers and others to appreciate the intrinsic and instrumental benefits of involvement and conduct involvement work in an inclusive and thoughtful way [19, 21]. The expectation that there will be public involvement across all aspects of health care research has been written into policy [36]. This embedding of public involvement in systems of health care and health research is an indication of its importance and the seriousness with which those in leadership positions take the need to include members of the public in important decision-making. Inclusion of the public has grown in the 24 years since the inception of INVOLVE, with involvement requirements starting with the patient-centered Research for Patient Benefit NIHR funding stream and moving across others in the NIHR portfolio. The new NIHR Centre offers opportunities for continued growth. It is unclear as yet the direction that will be taken or how the new systems will be developed, but this will unfold over the next few years and could lead to continued expansion in public involvement.

A centralized system for accessing information about public involvement and resources to support it is clearly beneficial. INVOLVE has played a leading role in evolving the conversation around public involvement and it is a trusted beacon of knowledge. PCORI also has a prominent role in providing national guidance on public involvement and leading the way to develop tools that support meaningful involvement. Although a centralized national source of knowledge has its benefits, such as easy accessibility and a principal and informed provider of advice, a potential downside could be the institutionalization of this knowledge. This could lead to the field maintaining a safer middle ground that is less easily challenged and advanced. The empowerment of INVOLVE's diverse Advisory Group including public members helped to counterbalance this risk.

An essential part of the work of INVOLVE has been its egalitarian approach to deciding on direction and developing resources. INVOLVE went to great lengths to ensure a diversity of perspectives existed within its advisory group, and members turned over regularly to allow new voices and ideas to be included. This transparent method of co-production was thoughtful and impressive, and it established a trusting and open atmosphere. This may also have engendered trust amongst the wider public, who could see public voices were included and impactful.

INVOLVE stimulated and facilitated a broad network of public contributors, public involvement facilitators, and researchers to build a culture of involvement in health and social care research. The biannual conferences provided a place for health professionals, researchers, and public members to come together, make connections, and discuss the field of public involvement in research. It was a unique event, attracting people from countries as far away Australia and the US to attend. This network complemented the structural embedding of involvement within the NIHR and led to local, regional, and organizational initiatives that continue to support public involvement on the ground (e.g. People in Health West of England [37] and Vocal [38]).

What Can We Learn Together?

Over the past few decades, England and the US have paved the way for meaningful public involvement in health research. A bibliometric analysis conducted to characterize the evolution of literature on public involvement in health research found that authors from the US and UK were the most likely to publish papers in this area. During the time period the authors studied, 1995 to 2009, they found that the numbers of empirical studies began to catch up with and then surpass literature reviews on public involvement in research, suggesting many more researchers were actively involving the public and writing about their experiences, even prior to the launch of PCORI in 2010 [2].

Broadly engaged team science is a newer concept, which marries the move toward transdisciplinary and multi-stakeholder work including researchers, clinicians, payers, industry, policy makers, and funders with the acknowledgement that communities and members of the public are important and essential stakeholders and must be included within teams. Broadly engaged team science is being conducted in creative and important ways, with Design Studios and Design Labs bringing multiple stakeholders together to brainstorm innovative solutions to health research challenges [39, 40]. Stakeholder mapping is being applied to health research, and people are seeing the benefits of thinking more broadly about stakeholders and bringing a widening group of perspectives to bear when conducting health research [20, 41].

Together we can think more inclusively, considering a broad variety of stakeholders and how best to empower them, supporting co-production of research as a team. Although both INVOLVE and PCORI have worked to support public involvement in health research, often this has meant partnership solely with health researchers, rather than wider teams of stakeholders. This expansion into other stakeholder groups will come with the potential for conflicts of interest and perspective. We can learn more about how to manage those conflicts, with a view to ensuring all voices are heard and recognizing that different perspectives will mean different pathways to solutions. It will be important to consider power imbalances and make sure a range of partners all have the support they need to interact and work productively together. Ensuring meaningful involvement of the public within broadly engaged team science will be essential. Researchers, public members, and others involved may need different tools and supports to contribute effectively, and these will have to be developed and iterated.

Approaches to Involving the Public in Health Research Continue to Evolve

England and the US have both established systems and structures to involve members of the public in health research as essential stakeholders with important perspectives. There are similarities and differences to their approaches, as we have outlined in this chapter. The important work that has been done to involve members of the public in health research is complemented by the idea of inclusive research teams moving towards broadly engaged team science. This concept is as context dependent as public involvement, and it will look different in different settings. We will need more time and further thought about how to meaningfully and actively involve an even wider range of stakeholders; however, the benefits will be a diversity of views and expertise on health care problems and solutions. We believe bringing stakeholders together to work creatively as a team and supporting public members to fully engage as research partners will improve the success of health research and its adoption into health practice.

References

1. NHS Executive Group (1995) Consumers and research in the NHS: an R & D contribution to consumer involvement in the NHS. NHS Executive, Leeds
2. Boote J, Wong R, Booth A (2015) Talking the talk or walking the walk? A bibliometric review of the literature on public involvement in health research published between 1995 and 2009. Health Expect 18(1):44–57. https://doi.org/10.1111/hex.12007
3. Department of Health (2007) Duty to involve patients strengthened: Briefing on section 242 of NHS Act 2006
4. NIHR National Institute for Health Research https://www.nihr.ac.uk/
5. NIHR Central Commissioning Facility (2019) Patient and Public Involvement and Engagement Plan 2019/20. https://www.nihr.ac.uk/documents/about-us/our-contribution-to-research/how-we-involve-patients-carers-and-the-public/CCF-PPIE-plan-2019-20.pdf
6. James Lind Alliance (2021) The James Lind Alliance Guidebook, version 10. Wessex Institute, University of Southampton, Southampton, UK. https://www.jla.nihr.ac.uk/jla-guidebook/downloads/JLA-Guidebook-Version-10-March-2021.pdf
7. Oliver S, Clarke-Jones L, Rees R, Milne R, Buchanan P, Gabbay J, Gyte G, Oakley A, Stein K (2004) Involving consumers in research and development agenda setting for the NHS: developing an evidence-based approach. Health Technol Assess 8 (15):1–148, III-IV. doi:10.3310/hta8150
8. Research Design Service (RDS). http://www.rds-sw.nihr.ac.uk/documents/NIHR-Overview-Document.pdf
9. Breaking Boundaries Review Team (2015) Going the extra mile: Improving the nation's health and wellbeing through public involvement in research. https://www.nihr.ac.uk/documents/about-us/our-contribution-to-research/how-we-involve-patients-carers-and-the-public/Going-the-Extra-Mile.pdf
10. Staniszewska S, Denegri S, Matthews R, Minogue V (2018) Reviewing progress in public involvement in NIHR research: developing and implementing a new vision for the future. BMJ Open 8
11. Hickey G, Brearley, S, Coldham, T, Denegri, S, Green, G, Staniszewska, S, Tembo, D, Torok, K, and Turner, K (2018) Guidance on co-producing a research project. National Institute for Health Research
12. National Institute of Clinical Excellence (NICE) Patient and public involvement policy. https://www.nice.org.uk/about/nice-communities/nice-and-the-public/public-involvement/public-involvement-programme/patient-public-involvement-policy
13. Barham L (2011) Public and patient involvement at the UK National Institute for Health and Clinical Excellence. Patient 4(1):1–10. https://doi.org/10.2165/11586090-000000000-00000
14. Elliott J (2013) HRA Strategy for Public Involvement NHS Health Research Authority http://www.hra.nhs.uk/documents/2013/10/hra-public-involvement-strategy-circulation-september-2013.pdf
15. Cancer Research UK. Patient involvement toolkit for researchers. https://www.cancerresearchuk.org/funding-for-researchers/patient-involvement-toolkit-for-researchers
16. British Heart Foundation. How you can help. https://www.bhf.org.uk/how-you-can-help/heart-voices. Accessed 13 May 2021
17. Wellcome Trust. How we engage the public. https://wellcome.org/what-we-do/our-work/public-engagement. Accessed 13 May 2021
18. Health Research Authority. What is public involvement in research? https://www.hra.nhs.uk/planning-and-improving-research/best-practice/public-involvement/
19. National Institute for Health Research (NIHR) Digital Strategy. https://sites.google.com/nihr.ac.uk/nihr-digital-strategy/home
20. PCORI (2014) Engagement Rubric for Applicants. http://www.pcori.org/sites/default/files/Engagement-Rubric.pdf. Accessed September 14 2020

21. Hanley B, Bradburn, J, Gorin, S et al (2000) Involving Consumers in Research and Development in the NHS: Briefing Notes for Researchers. Consumers in NHS Research Support Unit

22. Royle J, Steel R, Hanley B, Bradburn J (2001) Getting involved in research: a guide for consumers. Consumers in NHS Research Support Unit.

23. National Institute for Health Research (NIHR) (2020) NIHR launches new Centre for Engagement and Dissemination. https://www.nihr.ac.uk/news/nihr-launches-new-centre-for-engagement-and-dissemination/24576

24. NIHR INVOLVE Coordinating Centre INVOLVE Advisory Group - TERMS OF REFERENCE (2016). NHS National Institute for Health Research INVOLVE

25. NIHR (2021) INVOLVE. www.invo.org.uk

26. US Department of Health and Human Services. Director's Council of Public Representatives. FACADatabase.gov   https://www.facadatabase.gov/FACA/FACAPublicCommittee?id=a10t0000001h3NT Accessed November 2, 2020

27. The Patient Protection and Affordable Care Act (2010) Pub. L. No. 111-148, 124 Stat. 119

28. Patient-Centered Outcomes Research Institute (PCORI). About Us. https://www.pcori.org/about-us Accessed September 14, 2020

29. Patient-Centered Outcomes Research Institute (PCORI) Engagement. https://www.pcori.org/engagement Accessed November 2, 2020

30. INVOLVE response to the Department of Health Information Governance Review (2012). NHS National Institute for Health Research INVOLVE

31. Financial Compensation Of Patients, Caregivers, and Patient/Caregiver Organizations Engaged in PCORI-Funded Research as Engaged Research Partners (2015). PCORI Patient-Centered Outcomes Research Institute

32. Patient-Centered Outcomes Research Institute. Glossary. https://www.pcori.org/glossary. Accessed November 2, 2020

33. Richards (2017) Patient and public involvement in research goes global. The BMJ Opinion https://blogs.bmj.com/bmj/2017/11/30/tessa-richards-patient-and-public-involvement-in-research-goes-global/

34. Health and Social Care Act 2001 (2001) 15. United Kingdom

35. Evans D (2014) Patient and public involvement in research in the English NHS: a documentary analysis of the complex interplay of evidence and policy. Evidence & policy 10(3):361–377. https://doi.org/10.1332/174426413X662770

36. Department of Health (2006) Best Research for Best Health: Introducing a new national health research strategy.

37. People in Health West of England. http://www.phwe.org.uk/

38. Vocal. https://www.wearevocal.org/

39. Hirsch G, Trusheim M, Cobbs E, Bala M, Garner S, Hartman D, Isaacs K, Lumpkin M, Lim R, Oye K, Pezalla E, Saltonstall P, Selker H (2017) Corrigendum: adaptive biomedical innovation: evolving our global system to sustainably and safely bring new medicines to patients in need. Clin Pharmacol Ther 101(4):542. https://doi.org/10.1002/cpt.643

40. Hirsch G (2019) Leaping together toward sustainable, patient-centered innovation: the value of a multistakeholder safe haven for accelerating system change. Clin Pharmacol Ther 105(4):798–801. https://doi.org/10.1002/cpt.1237

41. Concannon TW, Meissner P, Grunbaum JA, McElwee N, Guise JM, Santa J, Conway PH, Daudelin D, Morrato EH, Leslie LK (2012) A new taxonomy for stakeholder engagement in patient-centered outcomes research. J Gen Intern Med 27(8):985–991. https://doi.org/10.1007/s11606-012-2037-1

Chapter 11
Leveling the Playing Field for Community Stakeholders: Examining Practices to Improve Engagement and Address Power Dynamics

Sara Folta, Linda B. Hudson, Beverly Cohen, and Apolo Cátala

Abstract Non-scientist community stakeholders ("community stakeholders") are an integral part of the translational research process. The knowledge they possess illuminates the social, political, economic, and cultural contexts from which participants and collaborators are drawn. In particular, the complex interaction of environment and history and their influence on the attitudes and perceptions of underrepresented populations should be understood, valued, and articulated in order to establish a meaningful relationship for all parties. However, this can only happen when those engaged in the research process understand and utilize effective strategies for community engagement and the management of power dynamics. In this chapter we explore approaches for expanding community engagement, including several strategies that use critical race theory as a framework for improving the equitable distribution of decision-making power. We also provide authentic reflections by members from each of our community-facing advisory boards, the Integrating Underrepresented Populations in Research Steering Committee and the Stakeholder Expert Panel, to highlight the community stakeholder perspective on the research process from inception to dissemination of results.

S. Folta (✉)
Tufts Clinical and Translational Science Institute, Boston, MA, USA

Friedman School of Nutrition Science and Policy, Tufts University, Boston, MA, USA
e-mail: sara.folta@tufts.edu

L. B. Hudson
Tufts Clinical and Translational Science Institute, Boston, MA, USA

Tufts University School of Medicine, Boston, MA, USA
e-mail: sara.folta@tufts.edu

B. Cohen · A. Cátala
Tufts CTSI Stakeholder Panel, Boston, MA, USA

© The Author(s), under exclusive license to Springer Nature Switzerland AG 2022
D. Lerner et al. (eds.), *Broadly Engaged Team Science in Clinical and Translational Research*, https://doi.org/10.1007/978-3-030-83028-1_11

Keywords Equitable distribution of decision-making power · Community stakeholder perspective · Community research advisory boards · Linguistic capital

Non-scientist community stakeholders ("community stakeholders") are an integral part of the translational research process. The knowledge they possess illuminates the social, political, economic, and cultural contexts that can be important to producing better research. In particular, the complex interaction of environment and history and their influence on the attitudes and perceptions of underrepresented populations must be understood, valued, and articulated in order to establish a meaningful relationship for all parties [1]. However, this can only happen when researchers understand and utilize effective strategies for community engagement and the management of power dynamics.

In this chapter we explore approaches for expanding community engagement, including several strategies that use critical race theory as a framework for improving the equitable distribution of decision-making power. We also provide authentic reflections by members from each of our community-facing advisory boards, the Integrating Underrepresented Populations in Research Steering Committee and the Stakeholder Expert Panel, to highlight the community stakeholder perspective on the research process from inception to dissemination of results.

Our Experience

The catchment area for Tufts Clinical and Translational Science Institute (CTSI) includes some of the most prominent medical schools, schools of public health, and research institutions in the United States, many of which have interests in authentic engagement with communities of need. To facilitate the sharing of resources available for the benefit of community health enhancement and research opportunities at these organizations, Tufts CTSI's Integrating Underrepresented Populations in Research program decided to begin with informational interviews with community-based organizations that had prior contact with the CTSI through its partners, Community Benefits offices, prior community-based research partners, and networks of staff. We refer to these organizations and agencies as "gateway organizations" because securing their agreement to explore the possibility of collaboration and/or partnership, or at least to co-convene community education activities, provides evidence of our presence and intent for community engagement. These gateway organizations included a local public health department, which is extremely active with several centers of health care excellence, faith-based organizations and coalitions, social and civic organizations, and prior research collaborators.

At this early stage, we recognized the importance of securing potential core collaborators, determining mutual needs for partnerships, and answering the key questions of trust and sustainability: Why are you here? Why now? What do you bring to the table? We also identified key strengths and challenges in this process. For example, we learned that staffing is critical and that a consistent full-time active presence is necessary to reflect our intentions. In addition, we found that identification of a particular niche helps to distinguish our work from the many other agencies and organizations functioning within the same catchment area.

In our case, we have the expertise and resources to provide training and education on research partnerships, specific content areas expertise (e.g., The Friedman School of Nutrition of Tufts University), and intramural grant funding through which tangible resources can be brought to bear on joint interests to jumpstart research. However, these elements may not be enough to facilitate the sharing of resources. Establishing compelling reasons to collaborate, identifying areas of interest, and developing mutually agreed upon principles of research practice are ineffectual if there is a lack of attention to community engagement and the intricacies of the power dynamic between community stakeholders and researcher communities.

Promising Practices for Improving Community Engagement in Team Science

Evidence-based practices for engaging community stakeholders have been demonstrated using methods drawn from community-based participatory research (CBPR), community-engaged research (CeR), participatory action research (PAR), among other frameworks [2–4]. For example, potential partners have been attracted and recruited using several different activities, including educational forums about the purpose and focus of the research, targeted community outreach, and using formative research to generate promotional materials that tap into community stakeholders' attitudes and knowledge regarding the research process while promoting understanding about their legal rights and protections, as well as the processes for disseminating research results.

Although there is a substantial evidence to support the involvement of community members in the latter stages of the translational research continuum, there are fewer models in the literature of strategic approaches to engage at the T0-T2 levels. One strategy, specifically designed for basic scientists and early-stage research, involves using a community-engaged research navigator (CEnR-Nav) as a liaison between basic researchers and community stakeholders [5]. The CEnR-Nav's responsibilities include working with scientist teams during research conceptualization to help create an environment that supports community-engaged research throughout study planning, implementation, and dissemination of results. In this model, currently being utilized at the Rockefeller University Center for Clinical and Translational Science, the collective expertise of the CEnR-Navs is designed to span the translational research continuum, facilitating activities to reach "in" to basic scientists and reach "out" to communities. The benefit of this approach is the development of an infrastructure that has the potential to be sustainable and cost-effective; however, successful engagement using navigators depends on several critical factors, including organizational leadership support, developing a process that "focuses on mentored partnerships skills," establishing tangible benefits for all partners, aligned aims, and aggressive identification of funding opportunities [4].

Another strategy for engaging community stakeholders in research partnerships is to establish community advisory boards or, more specifically, community research advisory boards (CRABs) that include community stakeholders as empowered collaborators integrated into the research process [5]. By developing a CRAB, investigators can establish partnerships that advance community members' understanding of the value of research and ensure that the members of the CRAB are included in research activities. CRABs can function as think tanks conceptualizing ideas for research, sounding boards reflecting community values, norms, and interests, and as co-advisors providing concrete recommendations to academic research institutions and research sponsors for developing and implementing community-engaged research teams [6]. The literature shows that preliminary investment in a CRAB can establish a cohort of partners committed to aligning the interests of the academic researchers with those of non-scientists [7]. However, as with the use of community-engaged research navigators, these community-engaged partnerships require time to become sustainable, funding resources to support capacity-building for both the community stakeholders and the research community, and one more element that is too often overlooked: an equitable distribution of decision-making power.

Approaches to Address the Equitable Distribution of Decision-Making Power in Team Science

Creating an equitable distribution of decision-making power in broadly engaged research teams is an essential but often overlooked challenge to sustaining community partnerships. Researchers from privileged groups may have the luxury of being unaware of these power dynamics and community stakeholders, based on experience, may assume that there is no will to address them. Even if they are aware, many researchers lack the ability and confidence to address these issues effectively. Critical race theory can help because it provides a useful framework for examining the common issues that arise when research team members are not attentive to power dynamics.

For example, one strategy to improve equitable distribution of decision-making power in team science is to re-think the way introductions are handled. Academics and clinicians typically introduce themselves by listing their positions after their name. This helps orient them to each other within a hierarchical system. An assistant professor knows how to react when introduced to a dean; a research coordinator knows the unwritten rules on how to act around anyone with the advanced degree. Those within colleges and universities are so immersed in this system and culture that it is automatic and unnoticed, like breathing air. Whenever awareness surfaces, academics and clinicians still tend to act in ways that maintain the structure. No matter the rank, there is at least some belief in the ability to climb the hierarchy. This is an example of the ways in which "schools…maintain the potential to emancipate and empower" [8].

At issue for broadly engaged team science is the effect that this form of introduction has on those outside of academic research institutions or organizations. Through a critical race theory lens, such introductions reinforce a hierarchy that is based on white elites. They start the conversation by valuing one type of knowledge, a type gained through access to data and the higher education needed to decipher it, that is less accessible to marginalized communities through the perpetuation of systems and policies rooted in racism. When researchers introduce themselves with their titles (e.g., doctor, professor, director, manager, and coordinator) the potential consequences are that it may:

- Highlight a system that often excludes marginalized communities from access to resources
- Reignite anger and frustration regarding this differential access to resources.
- Negate and devalue the forms of knowledge and power that community members bring to the interaction. These forms of knowledge may have been developed outside of the traditional educational system.
- Reduce the possibility for meaningful interactions that make best use of broadly-engaged team science.

Alternative strategies for introductions based on critical race theory offer potential solutions that help establish a foundation of trust and respect for all types of knowledge. Essential Partners, an organization dedicated to fostering meaningful conversations, describe their approach to introductions:

Introductions invite people to begin to tell their story – to be known in the ways they want to be known. For that reason, we think intentionally about what kind of question we ask for people to introduce themselves, to build connections, trust, relationship, and context. We lean toward stories, values, and shining moments – toward things that people might have in common. We lean away from rank, position, resume, and how long someone has been in the community [9].

Broadly engaged teams are encouraged to take this approach to introductions to start to acknowledge that all participants are both seekers of truth and members of communities. These introductions set the stage for true engagement. As an example, from our own work at Tufts CTSI, we constructed introductions based on the Essential Partners approach. Everyone was asked to state their name and to talk about a person who had inspired them to do the work that they do. Everyone was given a minute to think this through before responding. Participants spoke about family members, mentors, and early teachers and the lasting impact these people had made on their lives. This allowed us to connect on shared values around equity, justice, and serving others.

Beyond introductions, it is also important to develop strategies that help research teams acknowledge the wealth of knowledge, skills, and abilities that members from marginalized communities bring to the scientific discourse. Critical race theory suggests that privileged groups may tend to value only specific forms of knowledge and skills; the point is not that marginalized communities are lacking in these, but that they may also have other forms that are less valued. For instance, researchers tend to place faith in the power of data—that which can be obtained through a systematic process of observation and experimentation—while under-valuing other types of knowledge, including lived experiences [10].

Yosso suggests that marginalized communities nurture multiple forms of capital, including linguistic capital, familial capital, social capital, navigational capital, and resistant capital [8]. There are many different practical approaches research teams can employ to honor these forms of capital when conducting broadly engaged team science. For example, linguistic capital acknowledges the intellectual, social, and cross-cultural skills attained through the ability to communicate in more than one language [8]. While this type of capital should be acknowledged valued, research teams must be careful not to over-utilize community members as cultural ambassadors, expecting them to become accurate spokespersons for an entire culture. Also, even when the stated purpose for their participation is broader, multi-lingual members must not become relegated to a translator role. Rather, research teams can structure interactions so that multiple forms of communication are used, which is important to valuing the perspectives of marginalized community members, perspectives that are seldom heard by white researchers [10]. For example, in addition to discussions about data, team members may be encouraged to bring examples of art, photography, and music, or engage in storytelling related to the issue at hand. Per the *Framework for Community Engagement,* developed by the National Institutes of Health (NIH) Director's Council of Public Representatives, this can help to encourage diverse perspectives rather than just tolerating them [1].

Familial capital is another source of cultural wealth that is often unrecognized. Familial capital refers to a sense of community history and often involves a commitment to community well-being. It is related to social capital, a form of capital that has received more acknowledgment by the research establishment since it has been linked to health outcomes [11]. Consistent with the *Framework for Community Engagement* directive to develop an effective dissemination plan, a primary strategy that researchers can use to value these types of capital is to provide information and resources to community team members in ways that will facilitate their sharing of those resources within their communities. For example, a research team involving Dr. Folta conducted a study exploring the impact of selective eating on social domains among transition-age youth with autism [12]. The study team included a community stakeholder, an autistic person who works as a disability advocate. The paper from this study was recently published, and we are working with our stakeholder to translate findings into an accessible format so that people of all abilities can learn from it. Our stakeholder will then disseminate it through her networks.

Navigational capital "acknowledges individual agency within institutional constraints" [8]. Researchers need to both recognize the difficulty that marginalized communities have in navigating through racially hostile university and hospital systems and honor the skills they have developed to do so effectively. A simple but important action that research teams can take in this regard is to hold a meaningful proportion of meetings in community settings. For example, Drs. Hudson and Folta have collaborated for several years on the development and evaluation of heart health programming for African American women. The study team for one of our studies included a community stakeholder who is a registered dietitian with extensive experience working in African American communities. We deliberately held meetings at her place of employment or at a restaurant in one of the communities where she works. This also sent a message that we valued her time and expertise.

Resistant capital refers to "those knowledges and skills fostered through oppositional behavior that challenges inequality" [8]. This type of capital can be valued in the broadly engaged team science context through reconciliation activities. An example is the Racial Healing Circles project that was organized by the University of California Davis Clinical and Translational Science Center. In this project, a series of dialogues served to foster healing among academic and community partners by strengthening the ability to talk about race, culture, color, and class. At Tufts University, the Breaking the Silence series has brought in expertise and fostered conversations on topics that affect our community, including the impact of racial bias and weight bias on health and patient care. In 2020, the Tufts CTSI sponsored the fourth event in the series, on confronting exclusion in research.

Community Stakeholder Perspective

Successful engagement of, or relationship building with, community stakeholders is a function of several critical capacity-building components, including transparency in communication and decision-making, relevance of research direction to the populations of interest, and mutual respect evidenced by equitable decision-making processes. Those engaged in the research process across the translational spectrum (T1-T4) from biological and clinical research to social, behavioral, educational, and policy research can all benefit from understanding and utilizing principles of community engagement, most often defined as "the process of working collaboratively with and through groups of people affiliated by geographic proximity, special interests, or similar situations to address issues affecting the wellbeing of those people" [13].

In its *Framework for Community Engagement*, the NIH strongly recommends community stakeholder participation in the research process and articulates five tenets designed to help researchers create and sustain community engagement while also improving accountability and equity among team members. The five core principles are listed below, followed by sentiments expressed by members of our community-facing advisory boards when we asked them for their perspective on each facet of the model:

- **Definition and scope of community engagement in research.** "I want to be valued," a community stakeholder said. "I want to know what is going on… and how what happens is important to the process of research and discovery and me."
- **Strong partnerships**. As one community stakeholder told us, "…Not everyone is interested… but most have an interest at large… they are interested generally on how research impacts their community or their lives. Everyone comes with a motive…"

- **Equitable power and responsibility**. "[Researcher must be]... committed to creating a space where it is okay to ask questions," a community stakeholder suggested. "Cultivate an environment....where lay person comes up with an insight that helps with the research process...[they miss]...the value they would get by engaging the community. Particularly because the community is so vast...culture, education, language, economics."
- **Capacity building.** One of the community stakeholders we interviewed described it this way: "[I want]...the opportunity to understand and learn what the science [is] behind the decisions being made for me and generations after me.... so much of it is not readily available."
- **Effective dissemination plan.** "..Others have helped me, and I want to give it back to my community," a community stakeholder said. "[Communication]: crafting the story....what's in it for me....on-going communication.... people have to understand what research is and the value of their time and input...at the end of the day what can they expect to see as a follow-up....full circle don't snub people....[they] need to keep you in the loop..."

Conclusion

In summary, the value of engaging community stakeholders is no longer a question of "if" or "why," but "when," and "how." Our experience with community stakeholders is that they are experienced about engaging in research partnerships and eager to learn how their engagement will contribute to improved population health and meaningful research. Identification of the resources, both human and financial, to operationalize and sustain community stakeholder engagement is essential. Beyond tangible resources, it will be critical to acknowledge and address power dynamics to ensure meaningful engagement that is truly built on a foundation of mutual respect and trust.

As we continue with this work both in service to the stakeholder communities we serve and the research science community we represent, it is incumbent on us to consider that our work is grounded in our commitment to being a trustworthy research institution whose core values of equity, inclusiveness, and anti-racism will be evident and measurable in all of our activities. Those core values include the development of training opportunities for researchers in understanding how to create a trustworthy institution, in addition to exploring opportunities for non-scientist stakeholder to be engaged in an advisory capacity at the highest levels of our organization. Continuing to document the process of building trust relationships yielding joint projects with community partners and documenting the strengths and challenges of our community engagement activities is important for replicability and sustainability. The community engagement process, by its very nature, is iterative and grounded in co-learning processes which we will continue to use to provide guidance on research direction, recruitment and retention strategies, and effective dissemination of how the research emerging from our community/academic partnerships aligns with community health.

References

1. Ahmed SM, Palermo A-GS (2010) Community engagement in research: frameworks for education and peer review. Am J Public Health 100(8):1380–1387. https://doi.org/10.2105/ajph.2009.178137
2. Wallerstein N, Duran B, Oetzel JG, Minkler M (2017) Community-based participatory research for health: advancing social and health equity. San Francisco, CA: John Wiley & Sons
3. Balls-Berry JE, Acosta-Pérez E (2017) The use of community engaged research principles to improve health: community academic partnerships for research. P R Health Sci J 36(2):84–85
4. Baum F, MacDougall C, Smith D (2006) Participatory action research. J Epidemiol Community Health 60(10):854–857. https://doi.org/10.1136/jech.2004.028662
5. Kost RG, Leinberger-Jabari A, Evering TH, Holt PR, Neville-Williams M, Vasquez KS, Coller BS, Tobin JN (2017) Helping basic scientists engage with community partners to enrich and accelerate translational research. Acad Med 92(3):374–379. https://doi.org/10.1097/ACM.0000000000001200
6. Ortega S, McAlvain MS, Briant KJ, Hohl S, Thompson B (2018) Perspectives of community advisory board members in a community-academic partnership. J Health Care Poor Underserved 29(4):1529–1543. https://doi.org/10.1353/hpu.2018.0110
7. Stewart MK, Boateng B, Joosten Y, Burshell D, Broughton H, Calhoun K, Huff Davis A, Hale R, Spencer N, Piechowski P, James L (2019) Community advisory boards: experiences and common practices of clinical and translational science award programs. J Clin Transl Sci 3(5):218–226. https://doi.org/10.1017/cts.2019.389
8. Yosso TJ (2005) Whose culture has capital? A critical race theory discussion of community cultural wealth. Race Ethn Educ 8(1):69–91. https://doi.org/10.1080/1361332052000341006
9. Herzig M, Chasin L (2019) Fostering dialogues across divides. Essential Partners. https://whatisessential.org/resources/fostering-dialogue-across-divides
10. Bernal DD (2002) Critical race theory, latino critical theory, and critical raced-gendered epistemologies: recognizing students of color as holders and creators of knowledge. Qual Inq 8(1):105–126. https://doi.org/10.1177/107780040200800107
11. Rodgers J, Valuev AV, Hswen Y, Subramanian SV (2019) Social capital and physical health: an updated review of the literature for 2007-2018. Soc Sci Med 236:112360. https://doi.org/10.1016/j.socscimed.2019.112360
12. Folta SC, Curtin C, Must A, Pehrson A, Ryan K, Bandini L (2020) Impact of selective eating on social domains among transition-age youth with autism spectrum disorder: a qualitative study. J Autism Dev Disord 50(8):2902–2912. https://doi.org/10.1007/s10803-020-04397-4
13. Clinical and translational science awards consortium community engagement key function committee task force on the principles of community engagement (2011) Principles of community engagement second edition

Chapter 12
Conceptualizing and Developing a Theory of Stakeholder-Driven Community Diffusion

Erin Hennessy and Christina D. Economos

Abstract Community coalitions have been effective in addressing public health problems; however, there is little research on the mechanisms by which this occurs. Understanding the processes by which coalitions conceive, design, diffuse, disseminate, and/or implement interventions is a critical step to translate research findings into impactful community public health initiatives. We used systems mapping to understand and visualize how the Shape Up Somerville (SUS) intervention—a social change movement to prevent obesity through whole-of-community policy and environmental change—evolved over time and the factors contributing to its success. This analysis informed the development of the Stakeholder-driven Community Diffusion (SDCD) theory. The SDCD theory was conceptualized, operationalized, and tested in the context of childhood obesity and is now being applied to other public health problems. It is one step toward building rigorous, well-informed theories and methods to support broad stakeholder engagement.

Keywords Stakeholder-Driven Community Diffusion (SDCD) theory · Shape up Somerville · Romp & chomp · Community coalitions · Community coalition action theory

Community coalitions are partnerships usually between groups, which are formed to expand resources and solve social, political, economic, and community health problems [1]. Coalitions are often constellations of multiple organizations operating in different settings and sectors (e.g., education and child and family services, local business, city government), working collectively towards a common objective. Public health researchers and practitioners increasingly are seeking to collaborate with community coalitions to amplify the success of their public health prevention and promotion efforts [1–5]. For example, Shape Up Somerville (SUS), a social

E. Hennessy (✉) · C. D. Economos
ChildObesity180, Friedman School of Nutrition Science and Policy, Tufts University, Boston, MA, USA
e-mail: erin.hennessy@tufts.edu

© The Author(s), under exclusive license to Springer Nature Switzerland AG 2022
D. Lerner et al. (eds.), *Broadly Engaged Team Science in Clinical and Translational Research*, https://doi.org/10.1007/978-3-030-83028-1_12

change movement to prevent obesity, utilized a whole-of-community strategy which employs community engagement processes and implements multiple strategies to improve the health of a population defined by a geographical boundary [6]. The intervention strategies were designed in partnership with, and diffused through, a community coalition dubbed the SUS Task Force [7]. The SUS Task Force was formed from an initial group of local health professionals and community advocates to address nutrition and physical activity in the community; an issue highlighted by local data. A pilot grant was leveraged to identify key stakeholders, assess community needs and assets, facilitate discussions among academics and stakeholders, and develop a community organizing plan. The initial Task Force grew to represent a community-university collaboration consisting of a diverse set of multisector stakeholders. Eventually, federal funding was secured to launch the SUS study. SUS activities became the interventions in a landmark study that is one of the first to demonstrate that, compared to control groups, children living in the intervention community had a significant decrease in BMI z-scores (relative weight adjusted for child age and sex) one and two years after the intervention began [8–10]. Following the research period, SUS successfully became embedded into public health programming in Somerville and continues as a city-wide program with a project director and the ongoing work of local partners (see https://www.somervillema.gov/departments/health-and-human-services/shape-somerville) [11].

During a similar time period as the SUS study, another community-focused obesity prevention trial was conducted in Australia: the Romp & Chomp project, a community-based and communitywide multi-strategy obesity prevention project focused on changing policy, sociocultural, and physical aspects of early childhood environments to favor obesity prevention [12–14]. Romp & Chomp succeeded in achieving a significant decrease in overweight and obesity prevalence among young children in the intervention community relative to controls [12, 13, 15]. Like SUS, Romp & Chomp involved a community coalition to guide the adoption, dissemination, and implementation of strategies focused on achieving policy and environmental change.

Despite the number of publications about SUS and Romp & Chomp describing the main or secondary effects, specific intervention components, and other activities, none of the publications has fully described *how, post-study,* SUS or Romp & Chomp unfolded over time and what the community coalition's role was in achieving this change [8–10, 12, 13, 15–22].

We attempted to answer questions about the SUS diffusion process and the community coalition's role in that process and make progress toward the overall aim of developing a theory of community coalition influence [23, 24]. Our efforts suggest that an understanding of a public health problem in the community, combined with enthusiasm for and commitment to preventing the problem, will diffuse through stakeholder networks to the broader community and act as a catalyst for community change [23, 24]. Understanding the processes by which coalitions conceive, design, diffuse, disseminate and/or implement interventions is a critical step to inform public prevention efforts and impact research outcomes [25, 26]. The scientific literature on community coalitions underscores the critical role they can play in creating relationships, improving stakeholders' capacity to create change in their communities, and addressing challenges synergistically so the group is able to do more together than organizations could do working independently [27].

A Systems Mapping Approach

As part of theory-building and future hypothesis testing we used systems mapping, a qualitative systems modeling approach that looks at how variables interact over time and form patterns of behaviors across the system [28–30]. In the case of SUS, systems mapping was used to better understand and visualize how SUS evolved over time and to identify factors contributing to its success [31]. For example, variables were created to capture elements in the system that existed and interacted during the intervention period (e.g. school food, crosswalks, restaurant portions, community capacity), and we explored their role in influencing dietary and physical activity behavior and weight and obesity.

Systems maps have been used for decades for a range of undertakings including as the starting point for simulation modelling and to represent the diffusion of a public health intervention [32]. The SUS systems mapping process allowed us to: (1) move beyond communicating fragments or parts of the SUS community intervention to communicating the whole of SUS; (2) retrospectively describe and visualize the key interactions of how SUS was adopted, disseminated, implemented, and sustained over time; and (3) convey a system structure and the interrelationships that comprise SUS. At the time we conducted the systems mapping process, few public health interventions had been conceptualized using such a holistic approach. As a result of using this process, we uncovered the important and unique role that the SUS Task Force played in all aspects of the intervention and its sustainability, which warranted further research and hypothesis testing of the diffusion mechanism from SUS task force to the community. Moreover, like the SUS systems map, a systems map of Romp & Chomp was created to retrospectively understand the dynamics of project implementation, which highlighted the important role of collaboration and a similar type of community task force in achieving intervention outcomes [14].

The Stakeholder-Driven Community Diffusion (SDCD) Theory

Taken together, the SUS and Romp & Chomp interventions and respective systems maps, along with the extant literature, informed the development of the Stakeholder-driven Community Diffusion (SDCD) theory illustrated in Fig. 12.1 [4]. This theory addresses how a group of convened stakeholders, such as a community coalition, create community change. The theory postulates that an understanding of a public

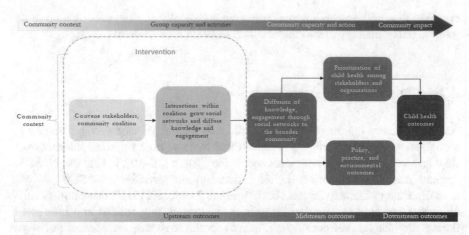

Fig. 12.1 The Stakeholder-driven Community Diffusion Theory and Theory-Informed Intervention. The Stakeholder-driven Community Diffusion theory and theory-informed intervention describes the hypothesized causal mechanisms by which knowledge and engagement of community coalition stakeholders diffuse across social networks within the coalition and out to the broader community, catalyzing change. Starting from the left, community context recognizes the critical role that the existing people, relationships, organizations, and ongoing work within a community play in determining the success of a coalition and coalition actions aimed to improve outcomes such as child health. Grounded in community context, the SDCD-informed intervention is designed to accelerate diffusion of knowledge and engagement, and growth in social networks through a set activities: (1) convening a multisector group of stakeholders to address child health; and (2) participating in Group Model Building activities to align the diverse perspectives of stakeholders, surface important systems insights about child health in the community, increase knowledge of and engagement around child health, and build new relationships; (3) prioritization of action strategies for intervention in the system, based on customized technical assistance for research evidence use and uptake; and finally (4) allocating project seed funding towards action identified by the group. This four-part intervention process is hypothesized to result in the diffusion of knowledge, engagement and research evidence use around child health through social network connections, into the organizations of the stakeholders who participate in the intervention. The resulting diffusion is hypothesized to increase the prioritization of child health initiatives among community decision-makers and organizations, which catalyzes and reinforces important policy, practice, and environmental improvements at the community level, which influence improved child health outcomes at the individual level

health problem in the community ("*knowledge*") combined with enthusiasm for and commitment to preventing the problem ("*engagement*") will diffuse through stakeholder networks ("*social networks*") to the broader community, hence acting as a catalyst for policy, practice and environmental change within the community [23, 24]. The SDCD theory has been conceptualized, operationalized and tested in the context of childhood obesity but has applicability to other complex public health problems.

The SDCD theory defines *knowledge* as "stakeholders' understanding of community-wide efforts to prevent childhood obesity" [33]. It consists of attributes identified from successful childhood obesity prevention interventions and drawn from existing measures such as the Community Capacity Index, the Community

Readiness Handbook, and the Community-based Participatory Research (CBPR) logic model [8, 12, 13, 34–37]. Within the knowledge dimension, five attributes include knowledge of: (1) the health problem; (2) modifiable determinants of the health problem; (3) stakeholders' roles related to addressing the problem in their community; (4) sustainable evidence-based intervention approaches to disrupt the problem (e.g. childhood obesity); and, (5) available resources.

The theory also posits that *engagement* motivates stakeholders to share their knowledge with others and represents stakeholders' desires and ability to translate their knowledge into effective action for community interventions [33]. It defines engagement as "stakeholders' enthusiasm for and commitment to preventing childhood obesity in their community" and includes five attributes: (1) exchange of skills and understanding ("Dialogue and mutual learning"); (2) willingness to compromise and adapt ("Flexibility"); (3) ability or capacity to affect the course of events, others' thinking, and behavior ("Influence and power"); (4) action of directing and being responsible for a group of people or course of events ("Leadership and stewardship"); and, (5) belief and confidence in others ("Trust") [33].

Social networks are networks of social interactions and personal relationships, and in the SDCD theory are defined as the network structure of stakeholders' professional relationships related to childhood obesity prevention efforts. Specifically, the number, strength, and influence of stakeholder social network connections represent the pathways for knowledge and engagement diffusion.

SDCD is informed by existing theories and frameworks from community psychology, and the multi-field science of diffusion and implementation science. These include the Community Coalition Action Theory and the CBPR conceptual model, which emphasize a lead agency or convener groups, member engagement, implementation of strategies, and the achievement of community change outcomes through coalition membership practices (*e.g.*, pooled resources, building capacity, implementing interventions and other strategies) [27, 35, 38, 39]. SDCD theory is aligned with recent reports that emphasize a focus on 'change agents' who can catalyze bottom-up demand and readiness for change [40].

Development and Testing of the SDCD Theory

Conceptualizing, designing, and testing the SDCD theory was possible through a groundbreaking five-year international collaboration to apply the principles of systems science to community-based childhood obesity interventions. The Childhood Obesity Modeling for Prevention and Community Transformation (COMPACT) study funded by NIH (R01HL115485). COMPACT was a multi-phased research endeavor that led to the creation of new tools to measure stakeholder engagement and techniques to understand the processes by which community coalition stakeholder groups influence outcomes. The study drew from our successful retrospective studies (SUS, Romp & Chomp) and included a prospective phase to test the theory in a new pilot study modeled after SUS but targeting a new population: children ages 0–5 years ("Shape Up Under-5").

Creating and Testing the SDCD Survey Tools and Mechanistic Model

To capture the key constructs of knowledge, engagement and social networks, we reviewed the literature on existing tools, but found weaknesses such as lack of detail on reliability and validity, narrow or limited domain areas, and lack of context specificity [33]. To overcome these limitations, we created a survey tool to measure the knowledge, engagement and social networks of community coalition members, which would then be used as the data inputs in our model.

We developed an agent-based model (ABM) to test the SDCD and understand whether and how knowledge and engagement of community coalition stakeholders (agents) diffuse through stakeholder social networks to the broader community. ABM is a computational tool that models the actions or interaction of 'agents' and allows for the exploration of dynamic mechanisms that link individual-level behavior to population-level outcomes [41, 42]. Several papers have addressed the rationale and advantages of applying ABM to the study of complex public health problems and interventions such as obesity [43–45]. ABM is well suited for diffusion models given its focus on individual-level interaction and its ability to capture social network structure mathematically. The ABM was initially built and tested using retrospective data from SUS and Romp & Chomp by testing the fit of simulated data to observed data. A combination of stakeholder survey data, intervention records, and expert estimates were used to populate the nascent model. Model output was evaluated against criteria derived from empirical data and experts' estimates of the magnitude and timing of community knowledge and engagement change. Details of results in Kasman et al. provide evidence of our hypothesis: increases in simulated community knowledge and engagement driven by SDCD closely matched expert estimates of magnitude and timing [24]. Model exploration also provided additional insights about these processes (including where additional data collection might prove most beneficial), as well as implications for the design and implementation of future interventions.

Following the retrospective phase, the ABM findings were applied prospectively to inform the design and evaluation of a pilot intervention, 'Shape Up Under-5' (2015–2017), to study the convening and dynamic processes of a community coalition working to prevent childhood obesity in children ages 0 to 5 years [23]. In brief, Shape Up Under-5 was a two-year early childhood obesity prevention pilot study in Somerville, Massachusetts (2015–2017) designed to test the SDCD theory. It involved a community coalition focused on addressing the issue of early childhood obesity that interacted during planned meetings held every four to six weeks throughout the study period.

To structure these meetings, we used Group Modeling Building (GMB). GMB is a participatory method led by trained facilitators who follow scripted, group exercises [46]. The process helps diverse stakeholders share their mental models (meaning their beliefs, assumptions and viewpoints of a problem) to visualize a complex and dynamic system, view connections across time and scale, and develop and prioritize action steps [47]. It has been cited as a promising approach for designing and adapting intervention strategies that take the inherent complexities into account [48]. In Shape Up Under-5, GMB was used to guide several meetings during the study period [49]. The use of GMB, a purposeful, planned and participatory technique, helped members to better understand the complex systems that influence problems of interest, take effective actions to address those problems, and equalize power among group members, enabling input from all participants and promoting group cohesion.

Eventually, the ABM will be extended to directly assess and connect the influence of the coalition on changes in policies, practices, and resource flows, and ultimately behavioral and biological changes in obesity. Details of the ABM, along with evidence supporting the SDCD as a key mechanism driving the success of a whole-of-community obesity prevention intervention are provided in Kasman et al. and forthcoming manuscripts [24].

Ongoing Research and Evaluation Efforts to Test and Refine SDCD Theory

Building from our SDCD theory, we have now designed and are testing the impact of an SDCD theory-informed intervention with five community coalitions across the US. (Cuyahoga County OH, East Boston, MA, Greenville, SC, Tucson, AZ, and Milwaukee, WI). The intervention encompasses three phases: (1) convene a group of stakeholders ("coalition") to identify important health trends and priorities in their community and explore the system driving those trends; (2) provide evidence-based strategies that align with coalition priorities, and (3) supply seed funding and technical support as the coalition works to implement and evaluate action(s). To begin, our team identifies 2–3 well-connected and impassioned community change-makers who are knowledgeable about complex drivers of health in their community. We work with them to identify and convene a multisector coalition to engage in participatory, structured group activities including GMB. The stakeholder group is intentionally drawn from different areas that impact children's health (e.g., education, food security, healthcare, public health, childcare, public policy, transportation, etc.).

As the coalition participates in structured group activities, stakeholders explore the complex relationships between drivers of health and gain insights about how to intervene in their community system to address those drivers. It is an iterative process; every subsequent session builds on outputs from the previous one. We intentionally share back the knowledge, engagement, and network data collected with the stakeholder group to guide their work and generate buy-in for sustained action and impact. An important outcome of the intervention, particularly within the stakeholder group, is the enhanced networking and capacity-building that arises from the regular meetings. While our social network data document the formation of relationship ties between stakeholders and community members in different sectors, we are also developing additional tools to capture the extent to which these ties form within the stakeholder group as a direct result of the meetings themselves.

Our research team supports the coalition's transition from exploration and understanding to action by sharing relevant evidence to inform their work, facilitating new partnerships to address they myriad social determinants that surface, and providing seed funding and technical assistance to guide successful implementation of evidence-based strategies. Ongoing research and evaluation efforts continue to test and refine our theory, and explore questions related to whether the SDCD-theory informed intervention improves outcomes among community coalition stakeholders involved in the intervention over time, and as compared community coalition stakeholders not involved in the intervention. Creation of a web-based data platform that harmonizes local data with our measurements and informs the strategic direction and investments of the community is also in development.

Connecting Upstream Influence to Downstream Outcomes

Community coalitions can be a powerful tool to amplify and diffuse public health prevention efforts that hold potential for reducing disease and improving population wellbeing. Elucidating the mechanisms by which these community stakeholders exert their influence can inform and improve public health interventions, yet there is scarce research on the mechanisms by which this occurs. Our efforts to develop and test the SDCD theory is one step toward building rigorous, well-informed theories and methods to support broad stakeholder engagement and realize the impact of community-based interventions. To build this new area of research, we turned to systems science, which has been well suited to address the inherent dynamic complexity of community coalitions. Initial testing provides suggestive evidence in support of our hypothesis that SDCD is a key driver of community coalition success. However, future research is needed to more rigorously assess and report on coalition involvement and to connect this upstream influence to downstream outcomes like child health. Our work offers an innovative approach to build and advance this field.

References

1. Butterfoss FD, Goodman RM, Wandersman A (1993) Community coalitions for prevention and health promotion. Health Educ Res 8(3):315–330. https://doi.org/10.1093/her/8.3.315

2. Butterfoss FD, Goodman RM, Wandersman A (1996) Community coalitions for prevention and health promotion: factors predicting satisfaction, participation, and planning. Health Educ Q 23(1):65–79. https://doi.org/10.1177/109019819602300105
3. Cormier S, Wargo M, Winslow W (2015) Transforming health care coalitions from hospitals to whole of community: lessons learned from two large health care organizations. Disaster Med Public Health Prep 9(6):712–716. https://doi.org/10.1017/dmp.2015.146
4. Korn AR, Hennessy E, Tovar A, Finn C, Hammond RA, Economos CD (2018b) Engaging coalitions in community-based childhood obesity prevention interventions: a mixed methods assessment. Child Obes 14(8):537–552. https://doi.org/10.1089/chi.2018.0032
5. Khan LK, Sobush K, Keener D, Goodman K, Lowry A, Kakietek J, Zaro S, Centers for Disease C, Prevention (2009) Recommended community strategies and measurements to prevent obesity in the United States. MMWR Recomm Rep 58(RR-7):1–26
6. Economos CD, Brownson RC, DeAngelis MA, Foerster SB, Foreman CT, Gregson J, Kumanyika SK, Pate RR (2001) What lessons have been learned from other attempts to guide social change? Nutr Rev 59(3):S40–S56. https://doi.org/10.1111/j.1753-4887.2001.tb06985.x
7. Chomitz V, Arsenault L, Garnett B, Hudson D (2013) Shape up Somerville: building and sustaining a healthy community. Shape up Somerville
8. Economos CD, Hyatt RR, Goldberg JP, Must A, Naumova EN, Collins JJ, Nelson ME (2007) A community intervention reduces BMI z-score in children: shape up Somerville first year results. Obesity (Silver Spring) 15(5):1325–1336. https://doi.org/10.1038/oby.2007.155
9. Economos CD, Hyatt RR, Must A, Goldberg JP, Kuder J, Naumova EN, Collins JJ, Nelson ME (2013) Shape up Somerville two-year results: a community-based environmental change intervention sustains weight reduction in children. Prev Med 57(4):322–327. https://doi.org/10.1016/j.ypmed.2013.06.001
10. Folta SC, Kuder JF, Goldberg JP, Hyatt RR, Must A, Naumova EN, Nelson ME, Economos CD (2013) Changes in diet and physical activity resulting from the shape up Somerville community intervention. BMC Pediatr 13:157. https://doi.org/10.1186/1471-2431-13-157
11. Economos CD, Curtatone JA (2010) Shaping up Somerville: a community initiative in Massachusetts. Prev Med 50(Suppl 1):S97–S98. https://doi.org/10.1016/j.ypmed.2009.10.017
12. de Groot FP, Robertson NM, Swinburn BA, de Silva-Sanigorski AM (2010) Increasing community capacity to prevent childhood obesity: challenges, lessons learned and results from the Romp & Chomp intervention. BMC Public Health 10:522. https://doi.org/10.1186/1471-2458-10-522
13. de Silva-Sanigorski AM, Bell AC, Kremer P, Nichols M, Crellin M, Smith M, Sharp S, de Groot F, Carpenter L, Boak R, Robertson N, Swinburn BA (2010) Reducing obesity in early childhood: results from Romp & Chomp, an Australian community-wide intervention program. Am J Clin Nutr 91(4):831–840. https://doi.org/10.3945/ajcn.2009.28826
14. Owen B, Brown AD, Kuhlberg J, Millar L, Nichols M, Economos C, Allender S (2018) Understanding a successful obesity prevention initiative in children under 5 from a systems perspective. PLoS One 13(3):e0195141. https://doi.org/10.1371/journal.pone.0195141
15. de Silva-Sanigorski AM, Bell AC, Kremer P, Park J, Demajo L, Smith M, Sharp S, Nichols M, Carpenter L, Boak R, Swinburn B (2012) Process and impact evaluation of the Romp & Chomp obesity prevention intervention in early childhood settings: lessons learned from implementation in preschools and long day care settings. Child Obes 8(3):205–215. https://doi.org/10.1089/chi.2011.0118
16. Coffield E, Nihiser AJ, Sherry B, Economos CD (2015) Shape up Somerville: change in parent body mass indexes during a child-targeted, community-based environmental change intervention. Am J Public Health 105(2):e83–e89. https://doi.org/10.2105/AJPH.2014.302361
17. de Silva-Sanigorski A, Elea D, Bell C, Kremer P, Carpenter L, Nichols M, Smith M, Sharp S, Boak R, Swinburn B (2011) Obesity prevention in the family day care setting: impact of the Romp & Chomp intervention on opportunities for children's physical activity and healthy eating. Child Care Health Dev 37(3):385–393. https://doi.org/10.1111/j.1365-2214.2010.01205.x

18. Economos CD, Folta SC, Goldberg J, Hudson D, Collins J, Baker Z, Lawson E, Nelson M (2009) A community-based restaurant initiative to increase availability of healthy menu options in Somerville, Massachusetts: shape up Somerville. Prev Chronic Dis 6(3):A102
19. Goldberg JP, Collins JJ, Folta SC, McLarney MJ, Kozower C, Kuder J, Clark V, Economos CD (2009) Retooling food service for early elementary school students in Somerville, Massachusetts: the shape up Somerville experience. Prev Chronic Dis 6(3):A103
20. Chomitz VR, McDonald JC, Aske DB, Arsenault LN, Rioles NA, Brukilacchio LB, Hacker KA, Cabral HJ (2012) Evaluation results from an active living intervention in Somerville, Massachusetts. Am J Prev Med 43(5 Suppl 4):S367–S378. https://doi.org/10.1016/j.amepre.2012.06.028
21. Burke NM, Chomitz VR, Rioles NA, Winslow SP, Brukilacchio LB, Baker JC (2009) The path to active living: physical activity through community design in Somerville, Massachusetts. Am J Prev Med 37(6 Suppl 2):S386–S394. https://doi.org/10.1016/j.amepre.2009.09.010
22. FSG (2013) Shape Up Somerville: A Collective Impact Case Study
23. Appel JM, Fullerton K, Hennessy E, Korn AR, Tovar A, Allender S, Hovmand PS, Kasman M, Swinburn BA, Hammond RA, Economos CD (2019) Design and methods of shape up under 5: integration of systems science and community-engaged research to prevent early childhood obesity. PLoS One 14(8):e0220169. https://doi.org/10.1371/journal.pone.0220169
24. Kasman M, Hammond RA, Heuberger B, Mack-Crane A, Purcell R, Economos C, Swinburn B, Allender S, Nichols M (2019) Activating a community: an agent-based model of Romp and Chomp, a whole-of-community childhood obesity intervention. Obesity (Silver Spring) 27(9):1494–1502. https://doi.org/10.1002/oby.22553
25. Sandoval JA, Lucero J, Oetzel J, Avila M, Belone L, Mau M, Pearson C, Tafoya G, Duran B, Iglesias Rios L, Wallerstein N (2012) Process and outcome constructs for evaluating community-based participatory research projects: a matrix of existing measures. Health Educ Res 27(4):680–690. https://doi.org/10.1093/her/cyr087
26. Gillman MW, Hammond RA (2016) Precision treatment and precision prevention: integrating "below and above the skin". JAMA Pediatr 170(1):9–10. https://doi.org/10.1001/jamapediatrics.2015.2786
27. Butterfoss FD, Kegler MC (2012) A coalition model for community action. In: Community organizing and community building for health and welfare. pp 309–328. doi: https://doi.org/10.36019/9780813553146-019
28. Foresight (2007) Building the obesity system map. Tackling obesities: future choices
29. Forrester JW (1964) Common foundations underlying engineering and management. SPEC 1(9):66–77. https://doi.org/10.1109/MSPEC.1964.6501138
30. Council. NR (2012) Accelerating progress in obesity prevention: solving the weight of the nation. The National Academies Press, Washington, DC. https://doi.org/10.17226/13275
31. Hennessy E, Economos CD, Hammond RA, Team SUSSM, the CT (2020) Integrating complex systems methods to advance obesity prevention intervention research. Health Educ Behav 47(2):213–223. https://doi.org/10.1177/1090198119898649
32. Greater than the sum systems: thinking in tobacco control (2007). NCI Tobacco Control Monograph Series 18
33. Korn AR, Hennessy E, Hammond RA, Allender S, Gillman MW, Kasman M, McGlashan J, Millar L, Owen B, Pachucki MC, Swinburn B, Tovar A, Economos CD (2018a) Development and testing of a novel survey to assess stakeholder-driven community diffusion of childhood obesity prevention efforts. BMC Public Health 18(1):681. https://doi.org/10.1186/s12889-018-5588-1
34. Edwards RW, Jumper-Thurman P, Plested BA, Oetting ER, Swanson L (2000) Community readiness: research to practice. J Community Psychol 28(3):291–307
35. Belone L, Lucero JE, Duran B, Tafoya G, Baker EA, Chan D, Chang C, Greene-Moton E, Kelley MA, Wallerstein N (2016) Community-based participatory research conceptual model: community partner consultation and face validity. Qual Health Res 26(1):117–135. https://doi.org/10.1177/1049732314557084

36. Lucero J, Wallerstein N, Duran B, Alegria M, Greene-Moton E, Israel B, Kastelic S, Magarati M, Oetzel J, Pearson C, Schulz A, Villegas M, White Hat ER (2018) Development of a mixed methods investigation of process and outcomes of community-based participatory research. J Mix Methods Res 12(1):55–74. https://doi.org/10.1177/1558689816633309

37. Oetzel JG, Zhou C, Duran B, Pearson C, Magarati M, Lucero J, Wallerstein N, Villegas M (2015) Establishing the psychometric properties of constructs in a community-based participatory research conceptual model. Am J Health Promot 29(5):e188–e202. https://doi.org/10.4278/ajhp.130731-QUAN-398

38. Stavor DC, Zedreck-Gonzalez J, Hoffmann RL (2017) Improving the use of evidence-based practice and research utilization through the identification of barriers to implementation in a critical access hospital. J Nurs Adm 47(1):56 61. https://doi.org/10.1097/NNA.0000000000000437

39. Gollust SE, Kite HA, Benning SJ, Callanan RA, Weisman SR, Nanney MS (2014) Use of research evidence in state policymaking for childhood obesity prevention in Minnesota. Am J Public Health 104(10):1894–1900. https://doi.org/10.2105/AJPH.2014.302137

40. Swinburn BA, Kraak VI, Allender S, Atkins VJ, Baker PI, Bogard JR, Brinsden H, Calvillo A, De Schutter O, Devarajan R, Ezzati M, Friel S, Goenka S, Hammond RA, Hastings G, Hawkes C, Herrero M, Hovmand PS, Howden M, Jaacks LM, Kapetanaki AB, Kasman M, Kuhnlein HV, Kumanyika SK, Larijani B, Lobstein T, Long MW, Matsudo VKR, Mills SDH, Morgan G, Morshed A, Nece PM, Pan A, Patterson DW, Sacks G, Shekar M, Simmons GL, Smit W, Tootee A, Vandevijvere S, Waterlander WE, Wolfenden L, Dietz WH (2019) The global syndemic of obesity, undernutrition, and climate change: the lancet commission report. Lancet 393(10173):791–846. https://doi.org/10.1016/S0140-6736(18)32822-8

41. Auchincloss AH, Diez Roux AV (2008) A new tool for epidemiology: the usefulness of dynamic-agent models in understanding place effects on health. Am J Epidemiol 168(1):1–8. https://doi.org/10.1093/aje/kwn118

42. Shoham DA, Hammond R, Rahmandad H, Wang Y, Hovmand P (2015) Modeling social norms and social influence in obesity. Curr Epidemiol Rep 2(1):71–79. https://doi.org/10.1007/s40471-014-0032-2

43. El-Sayed AM, Seemann L, Scarborough P, Galea S (2013) Are network-based interventions a useful antiobesity strategy? An application of simulation models for causal inference in epidemiology. Am J Epidemiol 178(2):287–295. https://doi.org/10.1093/aje/kws455

44. Hammond RA (2009) Complex systems modeling for obesity research. Prev Chronic Dis 6(3):A97

45. Sterman J, Rahmandad H (2008) Heterogeneity and network structure in the dynamics of diffusion: comparing agent-based and differential equation models. Manag Sci 54(5):998–1014. https://doi.org/10.1287/mnsc.1070.0787

46. Vennix JAM (1996) Group model building: facilitating team learning using system dynamics. J. Wiley, Chichester, New York

47. Carey G, Malbon E, Carey N, Joyce A, Crammond B, Carey A (2015) Systems science and systems thinking for public health: a systematic review of the field. BMJ Open 5(12):e009002. https://doi.org/10.1136/bmjopen-2015-009002

48. Burke JG, Lich KH, Neal JW, Meissner HI, Yonas M, Mabry PL (2015) Enhancing dissemination and implementation research using systems science methods. Int J Behav Med 22(3):283–291. https://doi.org/10.1007/s12529-014-9417-3

49. Korn A, Hovmand PS, Fullerton K, Zoellner N, Hennessy E, Tovar A, Hammond R, Economos C (2016) Use of group model building to develop implementation strategies for early childhood obesity prevention. 9th Annual Conference on the Science of Dissemination and Implementation in Health, Washington, DC

Chapter 13
Monitoring and Evaluation of Stakeholder Engagement in Health Care Research

Thomas W. Concannon and Marisha E. Palm

Abstract The landmark 2001 Institute of Medicine (IOM) *Quality Chasm* report called on the US. health care system to be based in shared knowledge, informed decisions, and patient-centeredness. In the nearly 20 years since the publication of the IOM report, there have been increases in the quantity and quality of stakeholder engagement, with newly developed frameworks supporting engagement throughout planning, conducting, and disseminating health care research. This chapter provides a roadmap to monitoring and evaluating post-Quality Chasm stakeholder engagement in health care research. We provide an overview of measurement domains and topics for the evaluation of stakeholder engagement in health care research. We distinguish between intrinsic and instrumental outcomes and make the case that both are essential to understanding the impacts of stakeholder engagement in research. We also recommend ways to report on the plans and results of evaluation work in research proposals, publications, and public communications. At the end of the chapter, we describe the major elements of a stakeholder engagement evaluation plan. Our intended audiences are funders of health research, research institutions, and research teams (including stakeholders) who may play important roles in future evaluation work.

Keywords Evaluation of stakeholder engagement · Stakeholder engagement evaluation plan · Engagement monitoring plan · Monitoring and evaluating engagement

T. W. Concannon (✉)
RAND Corporation, Boston, MA, USA

Tufts Clinical and Translational Science Institute, Boston, MA, USA
e-mail: tconcann@rand.org

M. E. Palm
Tufts Clinical and Translational Science Institute; Institute for Clinical Research and Health Policy Studies, Tufts Medical Center, Boston, MA, USA

© The Author(s), under exclusive license to Springer Nature Switzerland AG 2022
D. Lerner et al. (eds.), *Broadly Engaged Team Science in Clinical and Translational Research*, https://doi.org/10.1007/978-3-030-83028-1_13

Stakeholder engagement in health care research has its roots in conceptual models for community organizing [1]. Engaging communities in research emerged as a sub-discipline of health research over the course of the 1980s and 1990s with small federal investments in community-based participatory research and similar models. A hallmark of these models was the focus on engagement protocols that promote power sharing between researchers and community members.

The landmark 2001 Institute of Medicine (IOM) *Quality Chasm* report called on the US. health care system to be based in shared knowledge, informed decisions, and patient-centeredness [2]. This spurred many changes in health care delivery and research, including new authorizing legislation and research funding requirements for increased stakeholder engagement in health research [3–5]. The reforms introduced a fundamental shift in the health research field's conceptualization of stakeholder engagement. Whereas earlier community-based participatory research models identified stakeholders as interested parties from a defined geographic area, the new approaches identified stakeholders as decision-makers throughout the entire health care ecosystem [6].

In the nearly 20 years since the publication of the IOM report, there have been increases in the quantity and quality of stakeholder engagement, with newly developed frameworks supporting engagement throughout planning, conducting, and disseminating health care research [5, 7–9]. As the field matures, it is important to be able to measure how effective stakeholder engagement has been, including what impact it is having on health care research [10–16].

This chapter provides a roadmap to monitoring and evaluating post-Quality Chasm stakeholder engagement in health care research. We provide an overview of measurement domains and topics for the evaluation of stakeholder engagement in health care research. We distinguish between intrinsic and instrumental outcomes and make the case that both are essential to understanding the impacts of stakeholder engagement in research. We also recommend ways to report on the plans and results of evaluation work in research proposals, publications, and public communications.

At the end of the chapter, we describe the major elements of a stakeholder engagement evaluation plan. Our intended audiences are funders of health research, research institutions, and research teams (including stakeholders) who may play important roles in future evaluation work.

Monitoring and Evaluation Are Anchored in Engagement Aims

Plans for evaluating stakeholder engagement should align with the original intention and objectives of the study. For instance, if the purpose of engagement is to build a broader research community and to increase the quality of the research design by considering the areas of most importance to the stakeholders, these are the elements that should be measured for determining success.

The intrinsic value of stakeholder engagement is important; engaging stakeholders in a way that enhances their autonomy and dignity and allows their voices to be heard is often put forward as the right thing to do, especially given that the funds for health care research frequently come from public monies. It being the right thing to do means it is important that it be done well, hence the evaluation might measure how relationships have been built, autonomy has been maintained, and whether people feel their voices were heard. Until recently, much of the focus of evaluation of stakeholder engagement has been on intrinsic values like these.

Following the significant new investments in engagement work over the past two decades, many engagement advocates also call for evaluations that measure the instrumental impacts of engagement, such as its potential to make research more relevant, research methods more understandable, and research findings more useful.

Ideally, early in a project, researchers will have determined the purpose of the stakeholder engagement and will have incorporated measures of impact that will allow for the team to ensure that the aims of this activity are met. Reports on intrinsic evaluation have been useful to understanding what has worked to create a positive environment for stakeholder engagement [17]. More recently, reports of instrumental evaluation provide examples that stakeholder engagement positively affects research design, recruitment, study monitoring, and dissemination [8, 18, 19].

Monitoring and Evaluating Engagement

To date, approaches to monitoring and evaluating stakeholder engagement have been largely local and developmental in nature. Recent reviews point to the absence of shared governing frameworks, terminology and definitions surrounding home-grown approaches and to the absence of rigorous measure development, testing, and validation [15, 16]. In the interest of developing shared frameworks and terminology, we propose a simple but as-yet untested taxonomy that can help to set up a shared *engagement monitoring plan*. This taxonomy may serve as the basis for developing standardized monitoring topics.

Engagement work can be characterized according to a specific sequence of simple questions that both researchers and stakeholders will be familiar with: the who, what, when, where, how, why, and whether of engagement. Table 13.1 shows a potential way to group these questions into four domains: engagement content, context, process and outcomes. It also lists queries that would be useful to funders and research institutions who wish to monitor engagement, and research teams who want to evaluate the process and outcomes of their engagement.

Table 13.1 Engagement monitoring and evaluation domains and related topics

Domains	Related topics
Content	**Why** engagement is undertaken **Who** (which stakeholder communities) is engaged **Who** represents stakeholders **Who** initiates the engagement **What** is the intensity of engagement **What** research stages and activities involve stakeholders
Context	**Where** engagement is carried out **When** engagement is carried out
Process	**How** engagement work is carried out
Outcomes	**Whether** engagement meets its aims

Common Monitoring and Evaluation Topics

As discussed above, the reasons **why** researchers engage stakeholders—the aims of stakeholder engagement—can be described as either intrinsic or instrumental. Intrinsic aims may include whether the engagement process is authentic in that it that builds trusted relationships and allows stakeholders to fully participate in research teams [17, 20]. Instrumental aims may include strengthening the relevance of health research and ensuring research is better understood and incorporated into practice [2, 21–23].

Who is engaged, or which stakeholders are selected for engagement, can be described in reference to the stakeholder engagement taxonomies that have been developed, such as the 7Ps [7]. **Who** represents stakeholder communities may be important to understanding whether diversity, equity, and inclusion principles are being met. **Who** initiates engagement might also be captured; engagement can be researcher-initiated (as in most PCORI-funded research), partnership-initiated (as in Community-Based Participatory Research), or stakeholder-initiated (as in health advocacy movements like the 1980s and 90s AIDS Coalition to Unleash Power, or ACT-UP) [6].

What level or intensity of engagement is important to capture. This could be categorized using a recent adaptation of Arnstein's classic article introducing an eight-rung "ladder of citizen participation," which is today often referred to as the 4 Cs of engagement: communication, consultation, collaboration, and co-production [1, 24]. Stakeholders may be involved at different levels of intensity across activities. **What** research stages stakeholders are engaged in can be split into: preparing for, conducting, and using research. This can be further divided by activities within each of these stages, for example, using research could include peer reviewed publications, white papers, reporting, or presentations.

Where engagement is carried out should be recorded because place can easily be linked to and help shed light on community, language, and cultural influences. **When** engagement is carried out is also important for studying secular trends. Information about where and when stakeholder engagement takes place will provide funders with details that can help to explain how contextual information interacts with engagement processes or modifies engagement outcomes.

The processes around engagement, or **how** it is organized, can provide insight into what happened and whether it worked well for the researchers and other stakeholders engaged. Processes for recruitment, training, managing conflict, facilitation, modes, and roles of engagement can all provide information about how engagement was handled and what it looked like.

The outcomes of engagement circle back to the aims of the original why, and measure **whether** engagement has met the intrinsic or instrumental aims set out at the beginning of the research.

Developing an Engagement Monitoring and Evaluation Plan

As discussed above, the challenges associated with monitoring and evaluating engagement center principally on the absence of shared evaluation frameworks and measures. The focus of a monitoring and evaluation plan will depend on its intended audience(s) and objective(s). Researchers and stakeholders are often focused on evaluation that can help to improve engagement work, both in terms of how it is conducted and the impact that it has on the research and the individuals involved. Funders are likely to be interested in details of how stakeholders fit into research reporting, research teams, and institutions, as well as in the instrumental outcomes of engagement.

The steps for developing a stakeholder engagement evaluation plan include:

1. Discuss and clarify engagement aims with the study team, including stakeholders
2. Ensure that the plan aligns with study timing, budget, and other resources
3. Ensure that the plan focuses on aims agreed by the group
4. Agree on key indicators of success for each of the evaluation aims
5. Identify data that can be created or collected to address the key indicators
6. Use the data and indicators to monitor, evaluate and draw conclusions about engagement work

It is essential that stakeholder engagement evaluation results are shared with stakeholders and communities so that they can assess the value of ongoing involvement. It is also important that funders receive useful information that informs their approach to stakeholder engagement.

Metrics and Measures Will Continue to Evolve

Monitoring and evaluation of engagement in health research is an important part of building an evidence base and moving the field forward. We outline four distinct but complementary domains of evaluation: content, context, process, and outcomes, and list questions that align with each domain. The domains and questions contribute to building an overall picture of what stakeholder engagement work is comprised of, how it is being done, and what impact it has. As the field moves forward, it will be important to develop and validate metrics and measures that can be used by researchers to better understand the impacts of stakeholder engagement. The domains and topics, combined with the steps for building an evaluation plan, should help researchers who are involving stakeholders plan for evaluation early and think inclusively about how to measure the process and impacts of engagement.

References

1. Arnstein S (1969) A ladder of citizen participation. J Am Plan Assoc 35(4):216–224. https://doi.org/10.1080/01944366908977225
2. Institute of Medicine Committee on Quality of Health Care in A (2001) Crossing the quality chasm: a new health system for the 21st century. National Academies Press (US). Washington, DC, USA
3. Clinical and Translational Science Award U54 PAR-15-304 (2015) National Institutes of Health (NIH) https://grants.nih.gov/grants/guide/pa-files/par-15-304.html. Accessed 19 May 2021
4. About the CTSA Program (2019). https://ncats.nih.gov/ctsa/about. Accessed 19 May 2021
5. Sheridan S, Schrandt S, Forsythe L, Hilliard TS, Paez KA, Advisory Panel on Patient E (2017) The PCORI engagement rubric: promising practices for partnering in research. Ann Fam Med 15(2):165–170. https://doi.org/10.1370/afm.2042
6. Zimmerman EB, Concannon TW (2020) "Engaging Patients and Stakeholders in Health Research: An Introduction" in E. B. Zimmerman (Ed.), Researching health together: Engaging patients and stakeholders in health research from topic identification to policy change. Thousand Oaks, CA: SAGE Publishing, Mar 2020
7. Concannon TW, Meissner P, Grunbaum JA, McElwee N, Guise JM, Santa J, Conway PH, Daudelin D, Morrato EH, Leslie LK (2012) A new taxonomy for stakeholder engagement in patient-centered outcomes research. J Gen Intern Med 27(8):985–991. https://doi.org/10.1007/s11606-012-2037-1
8. Forsythe L, Heckert A, Margolis MK, Schrandt S, Frank L (2018) Methods and impact of engagement in research, from theory to practice and back again: early findings from the Patient-Centered Outcomes Research Institute. Qual Life Res 27(1):17–31. https://doi.org/10.1007/s11136-017-1581-x
9. Concannon TW, Grant S, Welch V, Petkovic J, Selby J, Crowe S, Synnot A, Greer-Smith R, Mayo-Wilson E, Tambor E, Tugwell P, Multi Stakeholder Engagement C (2019) Practical guidance for involving stakeholders in health research. J Gen Intern Med 34(3):458–463. https://doi.org/10.1007/s11606-018-4738-6
10. Barber R, Boote JD, Parry GD, Cooper CL, Yeeles P, Cook S (2012) Can the impact of public involvement on research be evaluated? A mixed methods study. Health Expect 15(3):229–241. https://doi.org/10.1111/j.1369-7625.2010.00660
11. Esmail L, Moore E, Rein A (2015) Evaluating patient and stakeholder engagement in research: moving from theory to practice. J Comp Eff Res 4(2):133–145. https://doi.org/10.2217/cer.14.79
12. Ray KN, Miller E (2017) Strengthening stakeholder-engaged research and research on stakeholder engagement. J Comp Eff Res 6(4):375–389. https://doi.org/10.2217/cer-2016-0096

13. Staniszewska S, Herron-Marx S, Mockford C (2008) Measuring the impact of patient and public involvement: the need for an evidence base. Int J Qual Health Care 20(6):373–374. https://doi.org/10.1093/intqhc/mzn044

14. Staniszewska S, Adebajo A, Barber R, Beresford P, Brady L-M, Brett J, Elliott J, Evans D, Haywood KL, Jones D, Mockford C, Nettle M, Rose D, Williamson T (2011) Developing the evidence base of patient and public involvement in health and social care research: the case for measuring impact. Int J Consum Stud 35(6):628–632. https://doi.org/10.1111/j.1470-6431.2011.01020

15. Boivin A, L'Esperance A, Gauvin FP, Dumez V, Macaulay AC, Lehoux P, Abelson J (2018) Patient and public engagement in research and health system decision making: a systematic review of evaluation tools. Health Expect 21(6):1075–1084. https://doi.org/10.1111/hex.12804

16. Bowen DJ, Hyams T, Goodman M, West KM, Harris-Wai J, Yu JH (2017) Systematic review of quantitative measures of stakeholder engagement. Clin Transl Sci 10(5):314–336. https://doi.org/10.1111/cts.12474

17. Wilson P, Mathie E, Keenan J, McNeilly E, Goodman C, Howe A, Poland F, Staniszewska S, Kendall S, Munday D, Cowe M, Peckham S (2015) Health services and delivery research. In: ReseArch with Patient and Public invOlvement: a RealisT evaluation – the RAPPORT study. NIHR Journals Library. https://doi.org/10.3310/hsdr03380

18. Brett J, Staniszewska S, Mockford C, Herron-Marx S, Hughes J, Tysall C, Suleman R (2014) Mapping the impact of patient and public involvement on health and social care research: a systematic review. Health Expect 17(5):637–650. https://doi.org/10.1111/j.1369-7625.2012.00795.x

19. Crocker JC, Ricci-Cabello I, Parker A, Hirst JA, Chant A, Petit-Zeman S, Evans D, Rees S (2018) Impact of patient and public involvement on enrolment and retention in clinical trials: systematic review and meta-analysis. BMJ 363:k4738. https://doi.org/10.1136/bmj.k4738

20. Johnson H, Ogden M, Brighton LJ, Etkind SN, Oluyase AO, Chukwusa E, Yu P, de Wolf-Linder S, Smith P, Bailey S, Koffman J, Evans CJ (2021) Patient and public involvement in palliative care research: what works, and why? A qualitative evaluation. Palliat Med 35(1):151–160. https://doi.org/10.1177/0269216320956819

21. McClellan M, Benner J, Garber AM, Meltze DO, Tunis SR, Pearson S (2009) Comparative effectiveness research: priorities, methods and impact. Brookings Institute

22. Draft National Priorities for Research and Research Agenda Version 1 (2012) PCORI Patient-Centered Outcomes Research Institute

23. Roehr B (2010) More stakeholder engagement is needed to improve quality of research, say US experts. BMJ 341(aug03 1):c4193. https://doi.org/10.1136/bmj.c4193

24. Crowe S (2017) Who inspired my thinking? – Sherry Arnstein. Res All 1(1):143. https://doi.org/10.18546/RFA.01.1.11

Part III
Applying Broadly Engaged Team Science: Case Studies

Chapter 14
Insiders and Outsiders: A Case Study of Fostering Research Partnerships Between Academic Health Centers and Corrections Institutions

Alysse G. Wurcel, Julia Zubiago, Deirdre J. Burke, Karen M. Freund, Stephenie Lemon, Curt Beckwith, John B. Wong, Amy LeClair, and Thomas W. Concannon

Abstract Hepatitis C is a blood-borne viral infection which can lead to liver disease and death. In 2013, an effective, well-tolerated, short-course oral treatment for hepatitis C was approved by the FDA. Despite widespread dissemination of curative hepatitis C virus (HCV) treatment in the community, HCV treatment in the corrections system has lagged behind with only 1% of people infected with HCV who are incarcerated in prisons and jails receiving treatment. A literature review revealed that most of the discussions about increasing HCV testing and treatment access in

A. G. Wurcel (✉) · J. Zubiago · D. J. Burke · A. LeClair
Tufts Medical Center, Boston, MA, USA

K. M. Freund
Tufts Clinical and Translational Science Institute; Boston, MA, USA

Department of Medicine; Tufts Medical Center and Tufts University School of Medicine
Boston, MA, USA

S. Lemon ·
University of Massachusetts Chan Medical School, Worcester, MA, USA

C. Beckwith
Alpert Medical School of Brown University, Providence, RI, USA

The Miriam Hospital, Providence, RI, USA

J. B. Wong
Tufts Clinical and Translational Science Institute; Division of Clinical Decision Making,
Department of Medicine, Tufts Medical Center, Boston, MA, USA

T. W. Concannon
RAND Corporation, Boston, MA, USA; Tufts Clinical and Translational Science Institute,
Boston, MA, USA
e-mail: awurcel@tuftsmedicalcenter.org

© The Author(s), under exclusive license to Springer Nature
Switzerland AG 2022
D. Lerner et al. (eds.), *Broadly Engaged Team Science in Clinical and
Translational Research*, https://doi.org/10.1007/978-3-030-83028-1_14

jails did not adequately reflect the views of crucial stakeholders—county sheriffs and correctional administrators. In this chapter, we discuss the development of partnerships with correctional administrators and the successful award of funding aimed at improving HCV testing and treatment access for correctional populations. We also describe the Stakeholder Framework we used in our research, as well as the lessons we learned in gathering these different perspectives.

Keywords Stakeholder framework · HCV care in jails · Health of correctional populations · HCV testing

Hepatitis C is a blood-borne viral infection which can lead to liver disease and death. In 2013, a highly effective, well-tolerated, short-course all-oral treatment for hepatitis C was approved by the United States Food and Drug Administration (FDA) [1]. Despite widespread dissemination of curative hepatitis C virus (HCV) treatment in the community, HCV treatment in the corrections system has lagged behind with only 1% of people infected with HCV who are incarcerated in prisons and jails receiving treatment in 2016 [2]. Based on literature review we concluded that most of the discussions about increasing HCV testing and treatment access in jails did not adequately reflect the views of crucial stakeholders—county sheriffs and correctional administrators. In this chapter, we discuss the development of partnerships with correctional administrators and the successful award of funding aimed at improving HCV testing and treatment access in jails. We also describe the Stakeholder Framework we used in our research, as well as the lessons we learned in gathering these different perspectives.

Correctional Health Care: A Brief History

One of the first jails[1] in the United States was built in 1690 in Barnstable County, Massachusetts with the original goals of providing punishment for crimes and improving public safety [3]. At the time, imprisonment was considered a more humane way of dealing with "offenders," in contrast to death or forced labor [4]. Currently, the United States incarcerates a higher percentage of people than any other country in the world and the vast majority of them are from populations that experience disproportionate barriers to health care (such as poverty, homelessness, and mental illness) [5, 6].

---

[1] Merriam Webster defines prisons as "an institution (such as one under state jurisdiction) for confinement of persons convicted of serious crimes" and *jail* is "such a place under the jurisdiction of a local government (such as a county) for the confinement of persons awaiting trial or those convicted of minor crimes."

In addition to their original goals, prisons are now also tasked with providing health care to those incarcerated; however, the American corrections system has a history of significant gaps in health care for people who are incarcerated. A survey conducted by the American Medical Association (AMA) in the early 1970s reported that only 6% of jail facilities performed medical examinations for all incoming inmates, more than 25% had no regularly scheduled physician visits, and 11% did not have available on-call physicians [7]. Then, the landmark *Estelle v. Gamble* case in 1976 found that deliberate indifference to a prisoner's serious illness or injury constitutes cruel and unusual punishment, leading to increased attention to ethical requirements for medical treatment and the creation of health standards for prisons [8, 9].

Collaboration between corrections administrators and medical professionals officially began in 1977, when the AMA held its first conference on improving correctional healthcare (now the National Conference on Correctional Healthcare) and published sets of health standards for prisons [9]. Around this time there was also heightened awareness about unethical research conducted in jails and prisons and the potential for coercion, and in 1978, the federal government severely restricted research on prison and jail inmates in medical studies [10–15].

The beginning of the HIV epidemic in the 1980s marked a crucial turning point for academic and corrections partnerships [7, 9, 16, 17]. Increased attention was directed toward the personal health of people who were incarcerated with infectious diseases, as well as the public health of the surrounding communities. Partnerships between departments of public health and corrections institutions were crucial for developing better case identification and treatment processes. The confluence of HIV and incarceration led to reexamination of the ethics of prohibiting people who are incarcerated from participating in research, since participation in HIV treatment research might extend their lives [18, 19]. During the height of the AIDS crisis, the median time from diagnosis to death from AIDS in people incarcerated in New York was 159 days, compared to 318 days for people not incarcerated [20]. Led by epidemiologists and public health professionals, these early research collaborations eventually extended to clinicians and researchers studying several diseases with high prevalence in the corrections system, including substance use disorder and HCV [21–27].

Collaborations that began as a result of HIV have opened some doors, but significant barriers to research about the health of correctional populations remain. For example, there is both limited funding for research in correctional institutions and complicated human subjects' protection policies. Such factors dissuade young investigators from research careers involving incarcerated populations. Our research team, led by Dr. Alysse Wurcel, found an opportunity for funding and worked with key stakeholders to partner in research aimed at understanding HCV testing and treatment policies in jails.

Developing a Partnership Between Tufts Medical Center and the Middlesex Sheriff's Office

When HCV medications were first approved in 2013, there were restrictions on HCV treatment based on severity of illness, and prior authorizations were required due to the high cost of the new medication. By 2015, insurance companies had relaxed these restrictions for the general population, based on an increase in treatment options and data to support treating people before cirrhosis developed. Treatment for HCV in jails and prisons, however, remained uncommon [28, 29].

When people are incarcerated, they lose their health insurance, and health care is provided by a pre-negotiated contract with health corporations. The high cost of HCV medications limits the feasibility of treatment for everyone who needs it [2, 29–31]. Since the 1970s "war on drugs," there has been a 600% increase in incarcerations—yet no commensurate increase in corrections healthcare budgets [5, 6, 32]. For example, modeling from Rhode Island (RI) estimated that treating all sentenced people for HCV would cost $17 million dollars, about six times the entire pharmacy budget for RI prisons [30].

Recognizing the opportunity for improving HCV care in jails, our team presented ideas for research on translating HCV care guidelines from the general population to the jail population at a March 2017 symposium at Tufts Medical Center, hosted by the Tufts Clinical and Translational Sciences Institute (CTSI). The special sheriff, superintendent and health services administrator from Middlesex County Sheriff's Office attended the presentation. The corrections administrators wished to partner on research to understand the best way to provide equitable access to treatment and address their concerns under increasing pressure to expand HCV treatment access in the jails.

With a solid commitment from the Middlesex Sheriff's Office and support from mentors, Dr. Wurcel received a two-year National Institutes of Health (NIH) Mentored Career Development grant from Tufts CTSI to assess perspectives of key stakeholders about barriers and facilitators to the HCV care delivery in jails. The goal of this research was to use mixed-methods (qualitative and quantitative) to address the gaps in knowledge around jail-specific HCV care. Previous qualitative literature on the topic of HCV care in corrections exists, but it is predominantly from prisons (not jails), international sites, or conducted prior to the current era of all oral, highly curative HCV treatments, and rarely includes non-incarcerated perspectives [33–39].

In order to capture a wide variety of perspectives, Dr. Wurcel used a framework known as the "7Ps" to identify stakeholder groups that play a role in HCV care decisions. The 7Ps stand for: (1) patients and the public: those who receive care, (2) providers of care (3) purchasers, who underwrite the costs (employers), (4) payers, who reimburse care (insurers), (5) policy makers, (6) product makers, such as drug manufacturers, and (7) principal investigators, or other researchers (Fig. 14.1) [40]. With support of the Middlesex Sheriff's Office, the research team identified and interviewed people who were incarcerated, corrections specialists, and clinicians

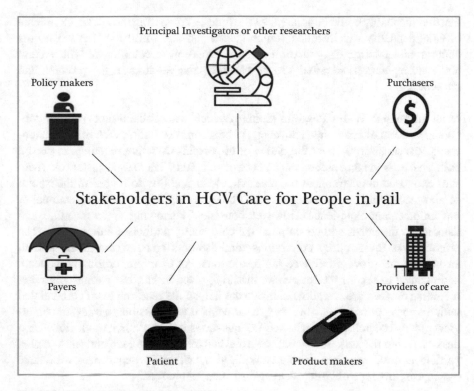

Principal Investigators or other researchers

Policy makers

Purchasers

Stakeholders in HCV Care for People in Jail

Payers

Providers of care

Patient

Product makers

Fig. 14.1 7Ps Stakeholder Framework [40]

and administrators who worked in the jail. Additionally, the team interviewed public health and policy representatives, people employed by pharmaceutical companies, and clinicians and administrators who worked outside of the jail but provided services for people with a history of incarceration. Gathering each of these perspectives shaped the results, ensuring they reflected a wide variety of barriers and facilitators to HCV care.

Lessons Learned

Build in Time for Institutional Review Board (IRB) Review. The IRB process for research involving people who are incarcerated requires more time and attention to confidentiality than research involving non-incarcerated populations. A prisoner representative was required to represent that perspective at IRB committee meetings, and while the IRB was able to recruit the prisoner representative, scheduling of IRB reviews was challenging and delayed IRB approval. Appropriately, there was intense scrutiny of the processes of recruiting people who were incarcerated, and the protocol needed extensive details to show that there was no coercion, and that confidentiality could be assured. As the funding came from the NIH, a Certificate of Confidentiality was awarded, which helped partially fulfill the IRB's concerns about confidentiality. Coordination of the submission in compliance with federal and state regulations required several meetings and versions of the protocol and consent form.

Meet In-Person When Possible Some research with collaborators can be conducted with email check-ins. However, the best communication with these collaborators was consistently over the phone or in-person. Attending meetings in-person built trust between the researchers and corrections staff. There were instances where staff expressed concern about the researcher team's ability to represent their point of view accurately because they "weren't blue," as in, did not have correctional or law enforcement experience. However, consistently showing up to meetings and listening to the needs and concerns of the community partners solidified trust. The protocol was reviewed by corrections administrators and lawyers at the jails to ensure that our process followed jail restrictions. For example, originally the team had planned to record the interviews that took place in jail, but phones and other recording devices are not allowed inside the jail, so the research team collaborated with the corrections administrators to ensure that it was possible to transcribe interviews (one research assistant asked the questions and the other transcribed on a desktop within the jail). Additionally, we had budgeted to give each non-incarcerated participant $50, but since people working at the Sheriff's department were state employees, any type of "gift" went against state regulations.

Researchers Need to be Accommodating There were logistical and timing challenges to reaching stakeholders who were incarcerated, or who worked at the jail. In order to enter the jail, each person on the research team was required to attend an orientation in the jail and have an escort when in the jail. Coordinating interviews with either group required near-daily communication with several different departments within the jail to determine appropriate times for research staff to enter the jail. While coordinating these interviews required more flexibility, more than half of the key stakeholders who participated in the study were incarcerated or worked in the jail. Our team reached out to about 100 people for interviews overall and completed 51 stakeholder interviews, including men who were incarcerated (patients, n = 21), clinicians working in jail and outside of jail (providers of care, and principal investigators, n = 12), corrections administrators (purchasers, n = 4), public health and policy representatives (n = 11), and people in HCV-related industry (payers, product makers, n = 3).

Continue to Engage Stakeholders in Analysis, Presentation, and Publication We made sure to communicate the results to our partners in the jail following initial analysis and to ask for feedback prior to submission of abstracts to conferences or any publications to journals. This is critical to ensure that our partners felt we represented their perspectives fairly. The interviews with key stakeholders identified both barriers to HCV care in the jails, and ways to improve HCV care. Some barriers to HCV care delivery included: (1) disparities in knowledge about HCV among people who are incarcerated, (2) transience of patients who are in jail, and (3) cost of HCV treatment. Opportunities for improved HCV care delivery included: (1) recognizing that when people are incarcerated the system can provide access to quality healthcare which may not be available in the community (2) testing for HCV in the jail setting and linking to care on the outside, and (3) negotiating payment methods to increase affordability of treatment in the jails. Our team has presented these research findings at international conferences, and we are preparing a manuscript for peer review.

Ongoing and Future Projects

The initial research partnership with the Middlesex Sheriff's Office has continued into ongoing research collaborations and a continued commitment to broadly engaged team science. This work has spawned a number of related research projects, such as a project aimed at using systems-science methodology to understand and improve HIV care transitions for people leaving jail and another aimed at assessing views of people who are incarcerated about different formulations of pre-exposure prophylaxis. Dr. Wurcel is collaborating on a study evaluating the impacts of making medication for opioid use disorder available in Massachusetts jails, including Middlesex County jail. She will be continuing to work with stakeholders from the jail on understanding and improving HCV-related care. In addition, Dr. Wurcel has been working closely with the Middlesex County Sheriff's Office in developing a COVID-19 prevention and mitigation plans for Massachusetts jails. A testament to the partnership, Middlesex County Sheriff, Peter Koutoujian, and Dr. Wurcel co-authored an Op-Ed in the Boston Globe, "State must ensure prisoners are protected against coronavirus," published March 23, 2020 [41]. The seeds of fruitful research were planted 4 years ago, and through open lines of communication, we are excited to continue to collaborate to improve infectious disease-care for correctional populations.

References

1. Barua S, Greenwald R, Grebely J, Dore GJ, Swan T, Taylor LE (2015) Restrictions for medicaid reimbursement of Sofosbuvir for the treatment of hepatitis C virus infection in the United States. Ann Intern Med 163(3):215–223. https://doi.org/10.7326/M15-04062
2. Beckman AL, Bilinski A, Boyko R et al (2016) New hepatitis C drugs are very costly and unavailable to many state prisoners. Health Aff (Millwood) 35(10):1893–1901
3. Massachusetts Cultural Resource Information System. http://mhc-macris.net/Details.aspx?MhcId=BRN.78
4. Barnes HE (1921) The historical origin of the prison system in America. J Am Inst Crim Law Criminol 12(1):35–60. https://doi.org/10.2307/1133652

5. Dumont DM, Gjelsvik A, Redmond N, Rich JD (2013) Jails as public health partners: incarceration and disparities among medically underserved men. Int J Mens Health 12(3):213–227. https://doi.org/10.3149/jmh.1203.213
6. Rich JD, Wakeman SE, Dickman SL (2011) Medicine and the epidemic of incarceration in the United States. N Engl J Med 364(22):2081–2083. https://doi.org/10.1056/NEJMp1102385
7. Glaser JB, Greifinger RB (1993) Correctional health care: a public health opportunity. Ann Intern Med 118(2):139–145. https://doi.org/10.7326/0003-4819-118-2-199301150-00010
8. (1976) Estelle v. Gamble. 429 U.S. 97
9. Reverby SM (2019) Can there be acceptable prison health care? Looking back on the 1970s. Public Health Rep 134(1):89–93. https://doi.org/10.1177/0033354918805985
10. Comfort N (2009) The prisoner as model organism: malaria research at Stateville Penitentiary. Stud Hist Phil Biol Biomed Sci 40(3):190–203. https://doi.org/10.1016/j.shpsc.2009.06.007
11. Hornblum AM (1999) Ethical lapses in dermatologic "research". Arch Dermatol 135(4):383–385. https://doi.org/10.1001/archderm.135.4.383
12. Protection of Human Subjects (2009). 45, vol 46. Office for Human Research Protections
13. Lerner BH (2007) Subjects or objects? Prisoners and human experimentation. N Engl J Med 356(18):1806–1807. https://doi.org/10.1056/NEJMp068280
14. Bach-y-Rita G (1974) The prisoner as an experimental subject. JAMA 229(1):45–46. https://doi.org/10.1001/jama.1974.03230390021016
15. Hodges RE, Bean WB (1967) The use of prisoners for medical research. JAMA 202(6):513–515
16. Farmer P, Campos NG (2004) Rethinking medical ethics: a view from below. Dev World Bioeth 4(1):17–41. https://doi.org/10.1111/j.1471-8731.2004.00065.x
17. Charles A, Draper H (2012) 'Equivalence of care' in prison medicine: is equivalence of process the right measure of equity? J Med Ethics 38(4):215–218. https://doi.org/10.1136/medethics-2011-100083
18. Collins A, Baumgartner D, Henry K (1995) U.S. prisoners' access to experimental HIV therapies. Minn Med 78(11):45–48
19. Dubler NN, Sidel VW (1989) On research on HIV infection and AIDS in correctional institutions. Milbank Q 67(2):171–207
20. Potler C (1988) AIDS in prison: a crisis in New York State corrections. Correctional Association of New York, New York
21. Dubler NN, Bergmann CM, Frankel ME, New York State AACAHCoAiCF (1990) Management of HIV infection in New York State prisons. Columbia Human Rights Law Rev 21(2):363–400
22. Vlahov D, Brewer F, Munoz A, Hall D, Taylor E, Polk BF (1989) Temporal trends of human immunodeficiency virus type 1 (HIV-1) infection among inmates entering a statewide prison system, 1985-1987. J Acquir Immune Defic Syndr 2(3):283–290
23. Dondero TJ Jr, Pappaioanou M, Curran JW (1988) Monitoring the levels and trends of HIV infection: the Public Health Service's HIV surveillance program. Public Health Rep 103(3):213–220
24. Binswanger IA, Stern MF, Deyo RA, Heagerty PJ, Cheadle A, Elmore JG, Koepsell TD (2007) Release from prison – a high risk of death for former inmates. N Engl J Med 356(2):157–165. https://doi.org/10.1056/NEJMsa064115
25. Springer SA, Qiu J, Saber-Tehrani AS, Altice FL (2012) Retention on buprenorphine is associated with high levels of maximal viral suppression among HIV-infected opioid dependent released prisoners. PLoS One 7(5):e38335. https://doi.org/10.1371/journal.pone.0038335
26. Kim AY, Nagami EH, Birch CE, Bowen MJ, Lauer GM, McGovern BH (2013) A simple strategy to identify acute hepatitis C virus infection among newly incarcerated injection drug users. Hepatology 57(3):944–952. https://doi.org/10.1002/hep.26113
27. McGovern BH, Wurcel A, Kim AY, Schulze zur Wiesch J, Bica I, Zaman MT, Timm J, Walker BD, Lauer GM (2006) Acute hepatitis C virus infection in incarcerated injection drug users. Clin Infect Dis 42(12):1663–1670. https://doi.org/10.1086/504327

28. Spaulding AC, Anderson EJ, Khan MA, Taborda-Vidarte CA, Phillips JA (2017) HIV and HCV in U.S. prisons and jails: the correctional facility as a bellwether over time for the community's infections. AIDS Rev 19(3):134–147

29. He T, Li K, Roberts MS, Spaulding AC, Ayer T, Grefenstette JJ, Chhatwal J (2016) Prevention of hepatitis C by screening and treatment in U.S. prisons. Ann Intern Med 164(2):84–92. https://doi.org/10.7326/M15-0617

30. Nguyen JT, Rich JD, Brockmann BW, Vohr F, Spaulding A, Montague BT (2015) A budget impact analysis of newly available hepatitis C therapeutics and the financial burden on a state correctional system. J Urban Health 92(4):635–649. https://doi.org/10.1007/s11524-015-9953-4

31. Sanger-Katz M (2014) Why the hepatitis cure Solvaldi is a budgetary disaster for prisons. The New York Times, p 3

32. Wildeman C, Wang EA (2017) Mass incarceration, public health, and widening inequality in the USA. Lancet 389(10077):1464–1474. https://doi.org/10.1016/S0140-6736(17)30259-3

33. Crowley D, Van Hout MC, Murphy C, Kelly E, Lambert JS, Cullen W (2018) Hepatitis C virus screening and treatment in Irish prisons from a governor and prison officer perspective - a qualitative exploration. Health Justice 6(1):23. https://doi.org/10.1186/s40352-018-0081-6

34. Khaw FM, Stobbart L, Murtagh MJ (2007) 'I just keep thinking I haven't got it because I'm not yellow': a qualitative study of the factors that influence the uptake of hepatitis C testing by prisoners. BMC Public Health 7:98. https://doi.org/10.1186/1471-2458-7-98

35. Ly W, Cocohoba J, Chyorny A, Halpern J, Auerswald C, Myers J (2018) Perspectives on integrated HIV and hepatitis C virus testing among persons entering a Northern California jail: a pilot study. J Acquir Immune Defic Syndr 78(2):214–220. https://doi.org/10.1097/QAI.0000000000001664

36. Lafferty L, Rance J, Grebely J, Lloyd AR, Dore GJ, Treloar C, Group ST-CS (2018) Understanding facilitators and barriers of direct-acting antiviral therapy for hepatitis C virus infection in prison. J Viral Hepat 25(12):1526–1532. https://doi.org/10.1111/jvh.12987

37. Jack K, Islip N, Linsley P, Thomson B, Patterson A (2017) Prison officers' views about hepatitis C testing and treatment: a qualitative enquiry. J Clin Nurs 26(13–14):1861–1868. https://doi.org/10.1111/jocn.13489

38. van der Meulen E (2017) "It goes on everywhere": injection drug use in Canadian federal prisons. Subst Use Misuse 52(7):884–891. https://doi.org/10.1080/10826084.2016.1264974. 40.

39. Yap L, Carruthers S, Thompson S et al (2014) A descriptive model of patient readiness, motivators, and hepatitis C treatment uptake among Australian prisoners. PLoS One 9(2):e87564

40. Concannon TW, Meissner P, Grunbaum JA, McElwee N, Guise JM, Santa J, Conway PH, Daudelin D, Morrato EH, Leslie LK (2012) A new taxonomy for stakeholder engagement in patient-centered outcomes research. J Gen Intern Med 27(8):985–991. https://doi.org/10.1007/s11606-012-2037-1

41. Wurcel A, Stone D, Koutoujian P (2020) State must ensure inmates are protected from coronavirus. Boston Globe

Chapter 15
Responding to the Community: HOPE (Healthy Outcomes from Positive Experiences)

Robert Sege, Dina Burstein, and Chloe Yang

Abstract Effective community-engaged research can provide powerful motivation and direction for the transformation of health care practice. In the case of the HOPE (Healthy Outcomes from Positive Experiences) project, we were able to translate research results into practice by engaging community members and stakeholders. In particular, we brought together a group of key individuals early in the process, which enabled the formation of a National Advisory Board (NAB) to help guide program development, leading to a strategic plan with broad stakeholder input. Our overall goal is to drive national adoption of the HOPE framework in clinical and community-based settings through a combination of education and practice transformation, advancing research, and community action. Our pathways to transformation include stakeholder engagement, shifting the narrative, changing practice, community action, public will building, and movement building.

Keywords Adverse childhood experiences (ACEs) · Positive childhood experiences (PCEs) · HOPE project

Effective community-engaged research can provide powerful motivation and direction for the transformation of health care practice. In the case of the HOPE (Healthy Outcomes from Positive Experiences) project, such research led to profound changes in how we interpreted and expanded knowledge, prompting the development of new clinical approaches that respond to the views of parents and families. As a result, the HOPE project is an example of translating research results into practice, as well as of engaging community members and key stakeholders in select aspects of the project development and dissemination process. The overarching goal of the project is

R. Sege (✉) ·
Tufts Clinical and Translational Science Institute; Center for Community Engaged Medicine, Tufts Medical Center, Boston, MA, USA

D. Burstein · C. Yang
Center for Community Engaged Medicine, Tufts Medical Center, Boston, MA, USA
e-mail: rsege@tuftsmedicalcenter.org

© The Author(s), under exclusive license to Springer Nature Switzerland AG 2022
D. Lerner et al. (eds.), *Broadly Engaged Team Science in Clinical and Translational Research*, https://doi.org/10.1007/978-3-030-83028-1_15

to promote the incorporation of a strengths-based, family-centric, and anti-racist approach into services directed at children and families. This new HOPE framework is rooted in both epidemiology and brain science, and its development and adoption by a diverse group of family-serving professionals illustrate many examples of strategies used in community-engaged translational research.

The objectives of this chapter are to: (1) describe the genesis of the ideas which led to the development of a new framework for care providers focusing on stakeholder involvement, and (2) discuss the ongoing process for stakeholder engagement and the continued development and broad implementation of HOPE.

The Complexities of Screening for Childhood Abuse, Neglect, and Dysfunction

The 1998 Adverse Childhood Experiences (ACEs) study demonstrated a dose-response relationship between 10 specific ACEs and adult health. These adverse experiences included child abuse, neglect, and family dysfunction. Adults who recall these childhood experiences have lower life expectancy and increased rates of a variety of physical and mental health problems [1].

Over the past decades, neuroscientists have explored the physical and anatomic correlates of ACEs. Jack P. Shonkoff, M.D., and his team at Harvard summarized and popularized these findings by coining the term "toxic stress" to encapsulate the physiologic changes linking ACEs with subsequent physical and mental health problems [2]. Based on powerful statistical associations between ACEs and adult health, ACEs screening has begun to move from public health surveys to the clinic. For example, Medi-Cal, the California Medical Assistance Program, began paying for ACEs screening in 2020 [3].

Despite widespread acceptance, the systematic incorporation of screening for adversity at the individual-level has created challenges for practitioners. For example, Ellis and Dietz noted that individual-level ACEs often resulted from underlying social and community issues, the roots of which are not necessarily solved at an individual-level [4]. Their model highlighted adverse community environments, including those resulting from systemic racism and historical trauma, that can lead to the abuse, neglect, and family dysfunction that formed the original ACEs in the 1998 study. Their paper pointed out the problems with turning systemic problems into individual ones and classifying individuals with a simple deficit score.

Other compelling data supported the importance of individual resilience, family strengths, and social and policy supports in optimal child development. For example, the Center for the Study of Social Policy in Washington, DC, developed and disseminated the Strengthening Families Approach™ to working with children and families, which focuses on five family-level protective/promotive factors that safeguard children from abuse [5]. These factors include concrete support in times of need, social connection, parental resilience and knowledge of child development, and the child's own social and emotional competence. As this strengths-based approach gained traction in child welfare and early childhood education circles, the ACEs study and concepts related to trauma-informed care came to be more widely accepted in health care.

Forming Research Ideas Based on Stakeholder Engagement

After meeting with frontline health and social service providers around the country, our perspective on ACEs screening changed, and we began to draw on a broader range of sources. For example, when one of the authors of this chapter (Dr. Robert Sege) participated in child abuse prevention meetings for local, state, and national organizations, he found that though the original ACEs questionnaire was not designed to be a clinical or diagnostic tool, many frontline workers knew their own ACEs scores [1]. In informal conversations at these meetings, it became clear that these providers were trying to make sense of their own lives while screening clients for their risks. Their own life experiences illustrated that the picture painted by an ACEs score was not determinative and often failed to provide actionable information about a family. In fact, it is common knowledge that many people, despite adversity, still manage to thrive [6, 7]. At one meeting, a provider who worked with teenagers aging out of the foster care system described how state-sponsored ACEs screening made teens feel doomed rather than hopeful because it failed to provide a full picture of their experiences with actionable steps forward. Another related how she and her colleagues spent their own time and money bringing young mothers and their children to playgrounds to play and have fun. This activity had to be hidden from management, which directed an evidence-based program focused on the identification of risks and referral to supports.

Inspired by these stories, we began to review the data and messages resulting from risk-based approaches to help us understand childhood experiences. Published data showed that many adults who suffered from ACEs escaped negative long-term physical and mental health consequences. For example, most (56%) adults who reported five or more ACEs do not suffer from depression [8, 9]. Dr. Christina Bethell at Johns Hopkins University shed light on this phenomenon, highlighting specific factors that lead to children's flourishing, even in the face of adversity [10].

Beginning in 2014, we sought to identify specific factors that explain how some adults avoid the expected consequences of ACEs. Together with The Montana Institute and the Wisconsin Department of Public Health, we added additional items to the population-based Behavioral Risk Factor Surveillance System (BRFSS) survey in Wisconsin [8]. These new items generated positive childhood experiences (PCEs) data and allowed us to compare health outcomes to the numbers of both ACEs and PCEs reported. Dr. Bethell led the analysis of these data. The results, first published as a monograph in 2017 and then in a peer-reviewed paper in 2019, clearly showed that specific PCEs could mitigate the effects of ACEs, supporting the idea of a PCEs score [11]. This approach validated community critiques that risk-factor screening results, on their own, are incomplete (and potentially misleading) assessments of individual patients and clients.

Listening to community critiques of common risk-based measures, including ACEs screening, led to the development of the HOPE framework, which describes four categories of positive childhood experiences needed for optimal child development. These are expressed as the four building blocks of HOPE; relationships with adults and other children; safe and stable environments with equitable opportunities to live, learn and play; social and civic engagement; and opportunities for social/emotional development [5]. This critical feedback, suggested by stakeholders in the field and explored by researchers focusing on people who thrive despite experiencing ACEs, was pivotal in leading our work in a new direction. The HOPE project has begun to attract national attention, even at this early phase.

We have successfully convened a National Advisory Board (NAB), which includes public- and private-sector leaders in pediatrics, child abuse prevention, home visiting, community development, and health equity. We created a HOPE website with an active blog and delivered numerous workshops and presentations to a variety of groups throughout the United States (Fig. 15.1). To date we have delivered over 50 presentations, webinars and workshops reaching over 10,000 individuals across the United States. Participants in our workshops have included frontline workers as well as policy makers from a wide variety of sectors including health care, home visiting, early childhood care and education, child protection and substance use prevention. We have reached physicians, nurses, government officials, social workers, home visitors and mental health professionals.

Over the coming years, the HOPE framework will be fully operationalized and widely disseminated. During this next phase of the project, we will be working toward the following objectives: (1) education and practice transformation; (2) advancing research by evaluating the impact of the HOPE framework on family and provider experiences; and (3) growing a HOPE-informed approach that identifies existing strengths and augments conditions that support the positive experiences children and families need to thrive. These objectives will require the development and dissemination of tools, materials, and resources to power the implementation of the HOPE framework and engage a growing community of practitioners. Additionally, we will provide training and technical assistance to organizations

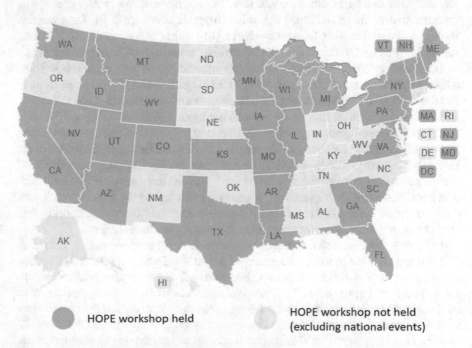

Fig. 15.1 Sites of HOPE training workshops 2020–2021

representing diverse sectors (health care, home visitation, early childhood education), populations served, and geographic locations to ensure the implementation of
the HOPE framework in their work.

Stakeholder Engagement in Strategic Planning

Stakeholder engagement is a key element in the strategic plan for implementing the
HOPE project (Fig. 15.2). To translate research findings into systemic changes to
trauma-informed care, we undertook the task of engaging a new set of stakeholders. Stakeholders for this work included parents and families, those who provide
services to them, and policy makers. To ensure that we had national reach with a
limited number of individuals, we identified organizations within each stakeholder
group, and then sought out individuals in leadership positions to advise us.
Throughout this process, we sought to maintain regional, racial, age, and ethnic
diversity.

In this planning phase, we focused on strategies consistent with our goal: widespread adoption of the HOPE framework in clinical and community-based settings.
Although many organizations and programs use strengths-based approaches, the
absence of an overarching, unifying framework precluded an integrated, holistic
view that incorporates knowledge of PCEs into established practice.

We identified four groups of stakeholders we planned to engage in the implementation and dissemination phase of our work:

1. Parents and children, particularly those who had experienced adversity
2. Pediatricians and other health care providers
3. Maternal/infant/early childhood home visitors
4. Policy makers and advocates

Systematic engagement of stakeholders began with the creation of the NAB. Some
of the organizations represented include: the Center for the Study of Social Policy,
Prevent Child Abuse America (PCAA), the New York Academy of Medicine, The
American Academy of Pediatrics (AAP) Section on Minority Health, Equity, and
Inclusion, and the Birth Parent National Network. Key consultants with expertise in
strategic planning, marketing and communications, and child health systems round
out the expertise available.

The main role of the NAB is to provide input and guidance on strategic planning and funding initiatives. Quarterly meetings are guided by agendas designed
to solicit strategic guidance. Board members further connect to additional key
stakeholders and decision makers through their own networks. Continual feedback from NAB members ensures the HOPE project is well-positioned to directly
engage with communities, parents, providers, and children in the future, making
it more likely that widespread implementation of HOPE practices will remain

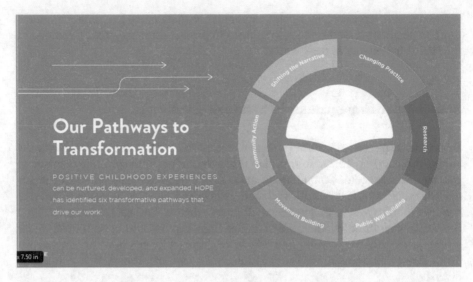

Fig. 15.2 HOPE pathways to transformation. HOPE seeks to catalyze a change in mindset among child and family service providers. The six strategic goals towards transforming the approaches taken are depicted in this graphic: Shifting the narrative from deficit-based to include strengths and resilience; changing practice towards collaborative problem-solving and away from the screen and refer paradigm; increasing the knowledge base through research; building public will through widespread engagement of local, state, and national leaders; building a movement through creating networking opportunities; and supporting community action to leverage the HOPE framework into policy changes [12]

relevant and useful to these stakeholders. HOPE National Resource Center staff call NAB meetings as needed and set the agenda. All board meetings are facilitated by an outside expert consultant.

Family-Centered Process Evaluation to Shape HOPE Project and Resources

Strategic planning included engagement with the Birth Parent National Network, a group of birth parents and organizations that engage parent voices to strengthen families, communities, and systems. In future, parent feedback will continue to shape the HOPE project and resources. Broader family input will be central to the implementation and dissemination of HOPE practices. To ensure candid and unbiased input, our independent evaluation team will design and conduct a family-centered process evaluation. Qualitative and quantitative techniques, interviews, and focus groups with parents and caregivers will be conducted to assess their experiences with HOPE-informed care. A HOPE family survey will be developed with the input of both practitioners and parents, forming a central component of ongoing evaluation and quality improvement.

Gathering Stakeholder Input from Public Health and Epidemiology Experts

In addition to the leadership advice provided by our NAB, the HOPE team specifically engaged the four important stakeholder groups mentioned earlier as we developed the strategic plan. The opinion of public health and epidemiology experts was sought through close collaboration with various health agencies and organizations, including:

Centers for Disease Control and Prevention We discussed HOPE with leadership and staff of the Division of Violence Prevention in the National Center for Injury Control and Prevention (NCIPC) at the CDC during an in-person visit that allowed us to present the research supporting the framework of HOPE, followed by several meetings and roundtable discussions with key leaders and staff. The NCIPC has appointed a liaison to the HOPE NAB, included HOPE items in their own national surveillance work, and provided funding for new surveys measuring PCEs in US families during the COVID-19 pandemic.

California ACES Connection On January 1, 2020, California launched a program to combat the negative effects of ACEs, the ACES Aware Initiative, spearheaded by California Surgeon General Nadine Burke Harris, MD. Through this program, the state now offers reimbursement for ACEs screening via Medi-Cal. The goal of these screenings is to identify individuals who have experienced ACEs, refer them to appropriate treatment, and reduce the long-term health effects. This program presented an ideal opportunity to incorporate HOPE into an important initiative as it is getting underway. The HOPE team, with the assistance of a California-based social impact strategy consultant, conducted a series of workshops to introduce the HOPE framework and garner feedback on how to integrate HOPE principles into the ACEs work in California. In February 2020, we conducted workshops in Sacramento and Long Beach and met with California ACEs Learning and Quality Improvement Collaborative (CALQIC) leadership in San Francisco, an 18-month long statewide learning collaborative that will oversee the implementation of ACEs screening in a group of pediatric and adult clinics in five different regions of California. Participants told us about tools and resources needed to speed this integration. We were enthusiastically received and have used our consultant report to develop strategic plans and relationships. Since that time, we have continued active partnerships with CA state agencies and coalitions. In 2021, ACEs COnnection changed its name to PACEs connection: Positive and Adverse Childhood Experiences, demonstrating the influence of the movement to consider the role of positive childhood experiences.

Prevent Child Abuse America PCAA is the nation's oldest and largest nonprofit organization dedicated to the prevention of child maltreatment. PCAA has a national network of state chapters, many of which also serve roles in state governments. Its home visiting network, Healthy Families America, is the country's largest home visiting model. Their deep knowledge of both family life and large-scale service delivery made them a clear partner for HOPE. In a virtual workshop with 15 staff members from PCAA and Healthy Families America, we presented the framework of HOPE and solicited their ideas and feedback on tools needed to move HOPE from research into practice. Participants were specifically queried on what tools and support they would need to integrate the HOPE framework into their work with families. Since that presentation, we have engaged with this organization and network to incorporate PCEs into their intake processes, and to develop new knowledge of PCEs and child abuse during the time of COVID-19.

American Academy of Pediatrics The AAP is committed to optimizing the mental, physical, and social well-being of all children. The AAP has significant reach and influence on policy and advocacy issues related to child health. We engaged with the AAP in several significant ways. The AAP currently has two representatives on the NAB, including the founding chair of the Section on Minority Health, Equity, and Inclusion at the AAP. HOPE is advising the AAP on messages concerning the effects of the COVID-19 pandemic on family life.

Engaging with these organizations is both an avenue for dissemination and a way to solicit feedback about the HOPE project, enabling us to continually make improvements and create the tools and resources different stakeholders need. In addition to the formal organizational partnerships described above, we have used ongoing interviews, blog posts, workshops, and webinars to promote bi-directional communication with key stakeholders. Developing and fostering authentic partnerships with key, influential stakeholders is critical to the development and dissemination of our novel framework.

Expanding Stakeholder Engagement for the Dissemination of HOPE

The next phase of the HOPE project is designed to move the project from innovation to implementation by early adopters, with the goal of influencing the majority of child- and family- service sectors within the next 3 years. This plan is built on the following strategic goals: (1) build broad awareness of the public health importance of PCEs, (2) stimulate interest in the HOPE framework for providers, frontline workers, and families, (3) draw out the HOPE framework's implications for key decision makers, including policy makers in organizations, institutions, and agencies, as well as philanthropists, and (4) engage a growing community of practitioners in the latest thinking and evidence on best practices to promote PCEs in clinical care.

Our strategic plan centers on continuous and meaningful engagement with the stakeholder groups that participated in planning, with increased involvement of parents and families as specific messages roll out. Focus groups with parents will elicit feedback on specific messaging and HOPE-related materials. This feedback will help us ensure that our parent-directed materials are acceptable, understandable, culturally appropriate, and useful.

The inputs to the strategic plan highlight continued attention to stakeholder engagement. In addition to input from the NAB and their organizations, parent and family input will be represented through a family-centered evaluation to be conducted by the Tufts Interdisciplinary Evaluation Research group. This evaluation will focus on family and child outcomes, assessing acceptability of the HOPE framework and parental perceptions of utility.

Activities and outputs of this process introduce a new network of multi-sector organizations and practices, the **HOPE Innovation Network**. This network of HOPE early adopters will help to support broad organizational change. The network will share periodic interactive webinars, implementation tools and resources, and strategies for implementing the HOPE framework. These organizations will form a learning community as they integrate HOPE into their work. Additionally, select organizations within this network will serve as case studies, allowing for an in-depth process and outcome evaluation of the HOPE framework.

Dissemination tools are currently included on the HOPE website, and we are now circulating a monthly newsletter [12]. The HOPE website serves primarily as a central hub for information and resources, disseminating materials, information, and results of implementing HOPE practices to key stakeholders. The website serves as the 'go to' place for practitioners from a variety of disciplines to learn more about PCEs and the HOPE framework. We continually update the website with content geared toward professionals in relevant fields (HOPE journal articles, worksheets, training webinars, and links to the online HOPE curriculum), and we feature items relevant to families and wider audiences.

The site also features the viewpoints of our stakeholders. NAB members and other nationally known professionals share this digital HOPE platform by writing guest blog posts or in published interviews, lending their expertise on topics ranging from health equity to child development, early relational health, and parenting in the context of COVID-19.

During 2020, the COVID-19 pandemic disrupted families and the provision of care for them. The HOPE National Resource Center provided training and technical assistance during this period. During the COIVD-19 pandemic, "[workshop] Emphasis was placed on parents' and providers' ability to both create positive experiences for children and reduce the anxiety and stress associated with the COVID-19 crisis and consequent stressors" [13].

We also reflected the lessons that we had learned from these workshops back to care providers. In early 2021, we published a reflection on our observations of family strengths and resilience during the pandemic [14].

Continued Engagement with Families and Communities

Engaging stakeholders was essential for every step in the development and dissemination of the HOPE project. HOPE arose from listening to community members' comments and critiques when discussing trauma-informed care. The development of the HOPE strategic plan relied on targeted outreach to key stakeholder organizations. Engagement of these stakeholders early in the design of the framework and development of the strategic plan has paid off, with continued investment in the development and implementation of HOPE.

Bringing together a group of individual and organizational stakeholders early in the process can help guide program development, leading to the creation of a strategic plan with broad stakeholder input. We used systematic in-person outreach through visits, workshops, and interviews to learn organizational perspectives and initially engage these partners, and we have carried this engagement through to the development of an NAB, in-person and virtual trainings, and an online presence. Each component provides opportunities for sustained engagement.

Continued engagement with enthusiastic stakeholders, including policy makers, practitioners, and parents and families, has been fundamental to ensuring the quality, relevance, and uptake of this project. We are committed to utilizing this strategy as we move the HOPE project forward.

References

1. Felitti VJ, Anda RF, Nordenberg D, Williamson DF, Spitz AM, Edwards V, Koss MP, Marks JS (1998) Relationship of childhood abuse and household dysfunction to many of the leading causes of death in adults. The Adverse Childhood Experiences (ACE) Study. Am J Prev Med 14(4):245–258. https://doi.org/10.1016/s0749-3797(98)00017-8
2. Shonkoff JP, Garner AS, Committee on Psychosocial Aspects of C, Family H, Committee on Early Childhood A, Dependent C, Section on D, Behavioral P (2012) The lifelong effects of early childhood adversity and toxic stress. Pediatrics 129(1):e232–e246. https://doi.org/10.1542/peds.2011-2663
3. Screening for adverse childhood experiences is a Medi-Cal covered benefit. (2020). ca.gov. https://files.medi-cal.ca.gov/pubsdoco/newsroom/newsroom_30091_02.aspx. Accessed 27 Feb 2021
4. Ellis WR, Dietz WH (2017) A new framework for addressing adverse childhood and community experiences: the building community resilience model. Acad Pediatr 17(7S):S86–S93. https://doi.org/10.1016/j.acap.2016.12.011
5. Sege RD, Harper Browne C (2017) Responding to ACEs with HOPE: health outcomes from positive experiences. Acad Pediatr 17(7S):S79–S85. https://doi.org/10.1016/j.acap.2017.03.007
6. Beckmann KA (2017) Mitigating adverse childhood experiences through Investments in early childhood pPrograms. Acad Pediatr 17(7S):S28–S29. https://doi.org/10.1016/j.acap.2016.09.004
7. Bethell C (2016) The new science of thriving. https://magazine.jhsph.edu/2016/spring/forum/rethinking-the-new-science-of-thriving/index.html/. Accessed 23 July 2020
8. Behavioral Risk Factor Surveillance System (2020). https://www.cdc.gov/brfss/index.html
9. Chapman DP, Whitfield CL, Felitti VJ, Dube SR, Edwards VJ, Anda RF (2004) Adverse childhood experiences and the risk of depressive disorders in adulthood. J Affect Disord 82(2):217–225. https://doi.org/10.1016/j.jad.2003.12.013
10. Bethell C, Gombojav N, Solloway M, Wissow L (2016) Adverse childhood experiences, resilience and mindfulness-based approaches: common denominator issues for children with emotional, mental, or behavioral problems. Child Adolesc Psychiatr Clin N Am 25(2):139–156. https://doi.org/10.1016/j.chc.2015.12.001
11. Bethell C, Jones J, Gombojav N, Linkenbach J, Sege R (2019) Positive childhood experiences and adult mental and relational health in a statewide sample: associations across adverse childhood experiences levels. JAMA Pediatr:e193007. https://doi.org/10.1001/jamapediatrics.2019.3007
12. HOPE (2021) Healthy outcomes from positive experiences. https://positiveexperience.org/. Accessed 02 May 2021
13. Burstein D, Yang C, Johnson K et al (2021) Transforming Practice with HOPE (Healthy Outcomes from Positive Experiences). Matern Child Health J 25:1019–1024. https://doi.org/10.1007/s10995-021-03173-9
14. Sege RD (2021) Reasons for HOPE. Pediatrics 147(5):e2020013987

Chapter 16
Students as Key Collaborators in Tackling Early Stage Research Ideas

Alissa Dangel and Mallory Whalen

Abstract When conducting collaborative research, emphasis is often placed on formulating a team of experts to address a specific challenge. However, some ideas are not yet ready for formal research. They represent early, undeveloped thoughts or the identification of a problem in need of a solution. Developing such early-stage ideas into a formal research project may provide an ideal opportunity to involve people who are not experienced researchers, but who nevertheless have skill sets that can be applied to brainstorming possible solutions. For example, students, who are often overlooked when formulating research teams because they are not yet "content" experts, can be effective for developing ideas, and eventually, for executing novel solutions to problems. In this chapter, we describe how a student-led team developed a prototype for a medical device designed to solve a specific clinical challenge: the prevention of head entrapment by an insufficiently dilated cervix in the setting of extremely preterm breech deliveries (less than 28 weeks of gestation). The project is in the pre-proposal stage and our goal is for the device to evolve to a point that a technology development grant proposal could be submitted and successfully funded.

Keywords Student-led team science · Collaborative research · Medical device design · Head entrapment · Breech delivery

When conducting collaborative research, emphasis is often placed on formulating a team of experts to address a specific challenge. However, some ideas are not yet ready for formal research. They represent early, undeveloped thoughts or the identification of a problem in need of a solution. Developing such early-stage ideas into a formal research project may provide an ideal opportunity to involve people who are

A. Dangel (✉)
Tufts Clinical and Translational Science Institute, Tufts Medical Center, Boston, MA, USA

M. Whalen
Dept of Mechanical Engineering, Massachusetts Institute of Technology, Cambridge, MA, USA

© The Author(s), under exclusive license to Springer Nature Switzerland AG 2022
D. Lerner et al. (eds.), *Broadly Engaged Team Science in Clinical and Translational Research*, https://doi.org/10.1007/978-3-030-83028-1_16

not experienced researchers, but who nevertheless have skill sets that can be applied to brainstorming possible solutions. For example, students, who are often over-looked when formulating research teams because they are not yet "content" experts, can be effective for developing ideas, and eventually, for executing novel solutions to problems. Their relative lack of exposure to strategies already in existence, or even to the problem itself, allows them to approach the concept from a fresh per-spective. In addition, many classroom and school-based environments typically encourage exploration and reward critical thinking, and a team-based approach to problem solving has become a specific focus for secondary and higher education [1].

A collaborative strategy that includes students can yield creative and potentially previously unrealized solutions to complex problems and/or identify important obstacles that need to be overcome in the design process. Scientists may not have access to or be aware of innovative education programs, like the one described in this chapter, that go beyond the usual internship experiences and instead are aimed at achieving successful collaborations between students and real world researchers. Such innovative programs provide students with the educational resources and sup-ports needed to ensure their collaborations with researchers succeed. In this chapter, we describe how a student-led team developed a prototype for a medical device that can be used to prevent head entrapment by an insufficiently dilated cervix in the setting of extremely preterm breech deliveries (less than 28 weeks of gestation). The project is in the pre-proposal stage and our goal is for the device to evolve to a point that a technology development grant proposal could be submitted and success-fully funded.

The Clinical Challenge: Prevention of Head Entrapment for Extremely Preterm Breech Deliveries

Vaginal delivery is typically avoided in extremely preterm breech fetuses due to the concern of head entrapment and as such, most extremely preterm breech deliveries are via cesarean. The national yearly average count for singleton extremely preterm breech deliveries derived from 3 years of data from the Center for Disease Control's National Vital Statistic Records (2016–2018) was estimated at 4,844. Of those, 87% (CI 86% – 88%) were delivered by cesarean [2]. In addition, at this very early ges-tational age, cesarean sections are frequently performed via vertical uterine inci-sions (classical) which produces additional associated maternal morbidity over horizontal incisions (low transverse), which are typically used at later gestational ages. Classical uterine incisions are associated with increased maternal morbidity, including the need for blood transfusions, compared with low transverse incisions [3–5]. Data from a large cohort study revealed that 53% of cesarean deliveries from 24 0/7 to 25 6/7 weeks were via classical cesareans, compared with 35% at 28 0/7 weeks and less than 10% at 35 0/7 weeks [6]. The subsequent risk of uterine rupture in a future pregnancy is also significantly elevated in patients with previous classical uterine incisions [7, 8]. This is despite a continued debate as to the neonatal benefits of cesarean delivery in this setting [9, 10]. One randomized clinical trial (RCT) to address this question, initiated in the 1990s, was stopped due to lack of recruitment [11]. Another RCT of extremely preterm breech vaginal delivery is unlikely to be conducted in the future. However, if head entrapment at the time of vaginal delivery could be prevented, a modified trial might become feasible.

Solving this problem is challenging on many fronts. First, there is little published data on the biomechanics of the human cervix in vivo or on head entrapment, and solutions need to address both the mechanical as well as the clinical aspects of this issue. Also, given that obstetrical complications, particularly one as specific as head entrapment, only affect a small number of people, there are limited resources from which to fund preliminary investigations.

Establishing a Non-traditional Multi-stakeholder Team

In order to initiate research and development on a very limited budget, a non-traditional approach to product development was needed. A brief announcement in a university newsletter seeking clinical challenges for students enrolled in a medical device design class offered a solution. It required no financial investment, only the investment of time and energy.

Medical Device Design, Course 2.75, at the Massachusetts Institute of Technology (MIT) provided a unique opportunity to establish a collaborative multi-stakeholder team to address the clinical challenge of preventing head entrapment [12]. This course pairs a group of students (senior undergraduate and graduate students in Mechanical Engineering) with a clinical advisor from academia or industry, and with faculty in the MIT Mechanical Engineering department to try to solve clinical problems [13]. Clinical advisors are encouraged to explain the problem thoroughly so that the students can conceptualize what type of solution might be appropriate and acceptable for that specific medical setting. Students are then free to brainstorm any number of possible solutions to the problem and receive feedback from the clinical advisors, their classmates, and the engineering faculty.

As shown in Fig. 16.1, a group of clinical advisors present the class with clinical challenges that have been vetted by engineering faculty. The students rank which projects they would like to work on. Students usually rank projects highly that they think are suited to their particular skill sets and pose intriguing problems. The course staff forms groups based on these rankings. The ranking and project selection process fosters a sense of ownership and responsibility in the students, likely more so than if they were randomly assigned to a project. Faculty members advise the projects that align with their areas of expertise. The class objectives are to go through the medical device design process and end with a proof of concept (T.0 or T.5) prototype.

The team assigned to the head entrapment project consisted of three senior undergraduates, one graduate student, one pre-doctoral teaching assistant, two engineering faculty mentors, and the clinical advisor. Figure 16.2 shows the contributions of each group to the team.

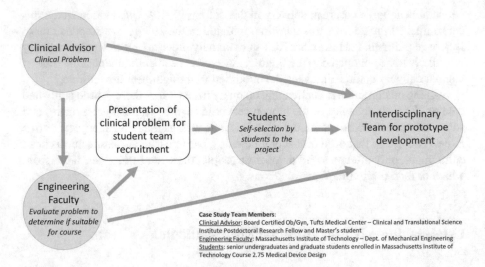

Case Study Team Members:
Clinical Advisor: Board Certified Ob/Gyn, Tufts Medical Center – Clinical and Translational Science
Institute Postdoctoral Research Fellow and Master's student
Engineering Faculty: Massachusetts Institute of Technology – Dept. of Mechanical Engineering
Students: senior undergraduates and graduate students enrolled in Massachusetts Institute of
Technology Course 2.75 Medical Device Design

Fig. 16.1 Team formation. The figure shows the process for team formation. The clinical advisor pitches the idea to engineering faculty who select the idea for their class. The students hear presentations for all the selected ideas and rank their top choices. Based on the rankings, the students are placed into groups and are paired with a clinical advisor and engineering faculty. The multi-stakeholder team members are as follows: Clinical Advisor: Board Certified Ob/Gyn, Tufts Medical Center – Clinical and Translational Science Institute Postdoctoral Research Fellow and Master's student; Engineering Faculty: Massachusetts Institute of Technology – Dept. of Mechanical Engineering; Students: senior undergraduates and graduate students enrolled in Massachusetts Institute of Technology Course 2.75 Medical Device Design

Research and Development of a Medical Device Prototype

None of the students, nor any of the other mentors except for the clinical advisor, had any personal experience with the proposed clinical problem. Weekly hour-long team meetings were scheduled to review any questions or concerns related to the clinical context and the engineering principles needed to develop a solution. These meetings provided a crucial opportunity for the team members to learn each other's "language" and appreciate the constraints of the respective settings. Key aspects of the clinical constraints needed to be clearly explained in everyday language to the engineering students since they did not have any experience with the Labor and Delivery setting. The clinical advisor explained clinical constraints by answering medical questions, providing educational material, participating in idea generation, and giving input on device manufacturing techniques and use of materials for patient care. As part of the weekly team meetings, the students provided updates on device design as well as how the materials themselves would influence subsequent iterations. Since the students had access to facilities where small-scale manufacturing could be done, they were able to test various options in real-time and provide this feedback to the clinical advisor. Knowledge from all these areas were shared under the larger umbrella of student-focused learning about the underlying engineering

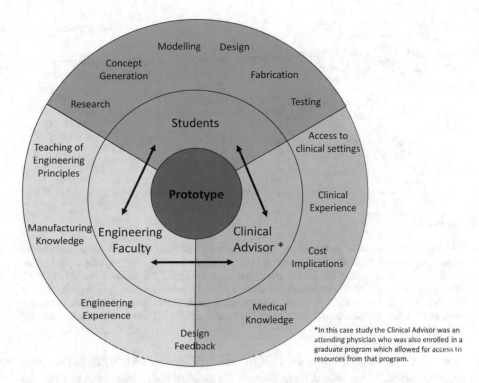

Fig. 16.2 The responsibilities of each group in the multi-stakeholder team

principles relevant to the design. The enhanced background information provided by the mentors to facilitate student learning also allowed for enhanced communication between the clinical advisor and the engineering team members. Figure 16.3 shows the flow of information and ideas among the team and between the team and other resources.

The students received a small monetary budget ($4,000) to purchase supplies, and over the semester, they designed several iterations of a prototype. Each iteration of the prototype was evaluated from both an engineering and manufacturing perspective, as well as for clinical appropriateness. This process was centered on the fundamentals of the deterministic engineering design process, which uses engineering principles to analytically characterize the product and minimize uncertainty [1]. By incorporating both the clinical and engineering mindset, potential device risks could be assessed from both perspectives. Weekly meetings allowed for rapid redesign if anyone from the team noted a problem with the design and assured that all necessary parameters were considered by the entire team. Students also had access to lab facilities and additional mentorship that allowed for supplementary input beyond that generated by core team members. For example, the students sought out an MIT faculty member who had done significant work modelling cervical properties. She was able to help them determine which of their device concepts would be most feasible. The students also gained access to an MIT lab that predominantly

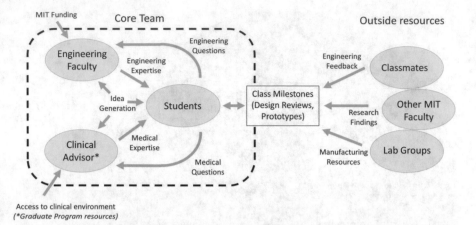

Fig. 16.3 Idea Review. In the core team, shown at left, expertise and ideas flow amongst the members. The students in the core team produce class milestones, such as design reviews and prototypes, that are evaluated by the outside resources, shown at right. The students use the feedback from the outside resources to improve upon their design with guidance from the other members in the core team. The team had a free flow of ideas amongst itself and leveraged outside resources, such as MIT faculty, who researched cervical properties, and a lab that had experience making inflatables

makes inflatable and soft devices. The students used the facilities in this lab to create their prototype. These interactions, along with those of their classmates working on other unrelated projects, provided a strong base for exploring numerous possibilities for device development.

Throughout the course, the team presented their progress as part of their structured curriculum. This allowed for additional feedback from their professors and classmates in a constructive manner. Further refinement of the prototype was made more efficient as a result of this information, and at the conclusion of the semester, a preliminary prototype of an expandable cervical balloon and retractor were completed [14]. The team also identified critical questions that need to be answered before the prototype could be tested in a clinical setting.

Student-Led Team Science Is a Valuable Resource for Solving Real World Clinical Problems

Successful medical device development requires a collaborative process and students can be valuable members of these teams. The initial step of connecting with students can be a potential obstacle but in this case was facilitated by personal connections, publicizing the MIT course outside of the direct university community via an alumni newsletter, and through cross-disciplinary academic partnerships. Members of the development team, the students, and their mentors were specifically allocated time to participate in all aspects of the course. This was further enhanced by the ability of the clinical advisor to also allot significant time to the project due to protected research time through a National Institutes of Health Clinical and Translational Science Awards (NIH CTSA)-sponsored fellowship. Additionally, this project benefitted from gaining a multidisciplinary perspective from its unique team of collaborators.

The physical setting of a university campus where the project took place (MIT) was also particularly important to the success of the project. Students reside in an environment that is conducive to exploration and novel idea generation. They are proximate to physical resources, such as machine shops and laboratories, and also to intellectual resources like professors and researchers. Although they are unpaid for their work, students are eager to pour themselves into these problems. They not only get to collaborate and learn from industry leaders, professors, and medical professionals but also get the chance to be involved in projects that will have significance outside of the classroom. Course-based student-led team science platforms provide an excellent foundation for addressing clinical challenges that may not be ready for scientific experts or attractive to industry involvement. Platforms like these enable students to participate in broadly engaged team science and help solve real world clinical problems.

Acknowledgements   Grant Numbers/Other Funding Source: Alissa Dangel, MD is a TL1 clinical research fellow funded by the National Center for Advancing Translational Sciences, National Institutes of Health, Award Number TL1TR002546.

Author's conflicts of interest: Dr. Alissa Dangel holds equity and consults for Mellitus, LLC. (Mellitus, LLC had no involvement in this project.)

References

1. Graham M, Slocum A, Sanchez RM (2007) Teaching high school students and college freshmen product development by deterministic design with PREP. ASME J Mech Des 129(7):677–681. https://doi.org/10.1115/1.2722334
2. Dangel A, Breeze J, Huggins G, House M, Kolandaivelu K (2019) 3096 estimation of the prevalence of cesarean delivery for the extremely preterm fetus in breech presentation. J Clin Translat Sci 3(S1):43–43. https://doi.org/10.1017/cts.2019.102
3. Patterson LS, O'Connell CM, Baskett TF (2002) Maternal and perinatal morbidity associated with classic and inverted T cesarean incisions. Obstet Gynecol 100(4):633–637. https://doi.org/10.1016/s0029-7844(02)02200-7
4. Kawakita T, Reddy UM, Grantz KL, Landy HJ, Desale S, Iqbal SN (2017) Maternal outcomes associated with early preterm cesarean delivery. Am J Obstet Gynecol 216(3):312 e311–312 e319. https://doi.org/10.1016/j.ajog.2016.11.1006
5. Luthra G, Gawade P, Starikov R, Markenson G (2013) Uterine incision-to-delivery interval and perinatal outcomes in transverse versus vertical incisions in preterm cesarean deliveries. J Matern Fetal Neonatal Med 26(18):1788–1791. https://doi.org/10.3109/14767058.2013.811226
6. Osmundson SS, Garabedian MJ, Lyell DJ (2013) Risk factors for classical hysterotomy by gestational age. Obstet Gynecol 122(4):845–850. https://doi.org/10.1097/AOG.0b013e3182a39731

7. ACOG Practice Bulletin No. 205: vaginal birth after cesarean delivery (2019) Obstet Gynecol 133(2)
8. Lannon SM, Guthrie KA, Reed SD, Gammill HS (2013) Mode of delivery at periviable gestational ages: impact on subsequent reproductive outcomes. J Perinat Med 41(6):691–697. https://doi.org/10.1515/jpm-2013-0023
9. Silver RM (2018) AGAINST: caesarean section is not the safest for extremely preterm breech. BJOG 125(6):666–666. https://doi.org/10.1111/1471-0528.15036
10. Carreno CA, Chauhan SP (2018) Caesarean section is the safest mode of delivery for extremely preterm breech singleton infants: FOR: caesarean delivery of extremely preterm breech singletons. BJOG 125(6):665–665. https://doi.org/10.1111/1471-0528.15037
11. Penn ZJ, Steer PJ, Grant A (1996) A multicentre randomised controlled trial comparing elective and selective caesarean section for the delivery of the preterm breech infant. Br J Obstet Gynaecol 103(7):684–689. https://doi.org/10.1111/j.1471-0528.1996.tb09838.x
12. MIT Medical Device Design Course. https://meddevdesign.mit.edu/. Accessed 28 Mar 2020
13. Hanumara NC, Begg ND, Walsh C, Custer D, Gupta R, Osborn LR, Slocum AH (2013) Classroom to clinic: merging education and research to efficiently prototype medical devices. IEEE J Transl Eng Health Med 1:4700107. https://doi.org/10.1109/JTEHM.2013.2271897
14. Whalen M, Chang-Davidson E, Moran T, Hoffman R, Frydman GH, Slocum A, Dangel A (2021) Device prototype for vaginal delivery of extremely preterm fetuses in the breech presentation. J Med Device 15(2):021002. https://doi.org/10.1115/1.4049086

Chapter 17
Engaging Stakeholders to Decrease Study Start-Up Delays

Denise H. Daudelin, Alyssa Cabrera, Alicea Riley, and Jaime Chisholm

Abstract The efficient study start-up of cancer clinical trials relies on coordinating the actions of a broad group of research staff and stakeholders. Unnecessary delays waste valuable research dollars and delay enrolling patients into potentially lifesaving studies. The Neely Center for Clinical Cancer Research (NCCCR) at Tufts Medical Center and Tufts Children's Hospital sought to identify and resolve study start-up delays that interfere with clinical trial activation and patient enrollment in industry-sponsored studies. Together with the Center for Research Process Improvement (CRPI) at Tufts Clinical and Translational Science Institute (CTSI), the NCCCR conducted a quality improvement effort to identify and resolve the causes of study start-up delays by engaging staff who best understand and are empowered to resolve those delays. The project led to the development of a study start-up toolkit that describes each step in the clinical trial activation process and includes background information, detailed instructions, and links to all resource materials and relevant individuals by role.

Keywords Causes of study start-up delays · Clinical trial activation · Study start-up · Study start-up toolkit · Quality improvement

The efficient study start-up of cancer clinical trials relies on coordinating the actions of a broad group of research staff and stakeholders. Study start-up procedures are often complex and challenging for staff to navigate, leading to unnecessary delays. These setbacks waste valuable research dollars and delay enrolling patients into

D. H. Daudelin (✉)
Tufts Clinical and Translational Science Institute; Institute for Clinical Research and Health Policy Studies, Tufts Medical Center, Boston, MA, USA

A. Cabrera · A. Riley
Tufts Clinical and Translational Science Institute; Tufts Medical Center, Boston, MA, USA

J. Chisholm
Tufts Medical Center, Boston, MA, USA
e-mail: ddaudelin@tuftsmedicalcenter.org

© The Author(s), under exclusive license to Springer Nature
Switzerland AG 2022
D. Lerner et al. (eds.), *Broadly Engaged Team Science in Clinical and Translational Research*, https://doi.org/10.1007/978-3-030-83028-1_17

potentially lifesaving studies [1]. The Neely Center for Clinical Cancer Research (NCCCR) at Tufts Medical Center and Tufts Children's Hospital sought to identify and resolve study start-up delays that interfere with clinical trial activation and patient enrollment in industry-sponsored studies. Together with the Center for Research Process Improvement (CRPI) at Tufts Clinical and Translational Science Institute (CTSI), the NCCCR conducted a quality improvement (QI) effort to identify and resolve the causes of study start-up delays by engaging staff who best understand and are empowered to resolve those delays [2].

Tufts CTSI created the CRPI to help researchers and research administration staff address research roadblocks using quality improvement methods. However, literature on the use of QI methods to improve clinical research in academic settings is limited [3, 4]. In health care, QI is defined as a structured organizational process for involving personnel in planning and executing a continuous flow of improvement to provide quality health care that meets or exceeds expectations [5]. Like health care, clinical research is conducted by individuals and teams working within organizational systems that may not always promote efficient, effective, and safe research processes and outcomes. The use of QI methods in clinical research—which we refer to as research process improvement (RPI)—can address both research system-level and study-level barriers to support the successful completion of clinical studies. The primary goals of the CRPI are to use these methods to improve the conduct of research throughout Tufts CTSI and its partner organizations and to build the capacity of researchers to integrate these methods within their own studies to foster a process of continuous improvement.

The CRPI team includes staff with experience in using QI methods in diverse health care and public health settings as well as in conducting clinical research. A team-based approach is used to advance the quality and efficiency of clinical research across the entire project duration, including:

- identifying an important problem
- engaging a robust team
- understanding the related processes
- determining underlying causes of delay and inefficiency
- developing and implementing change strategies
- measuring progress

This chapter describes a team-based research process improvement project to address delays in study start-up conducted by the NCCCR in conjunction with the CRPI team.

Identifying the Problem and Engaging the Team

The NCCCR strives to improve operational efficiency in cancer clinical trials, while maintaining the current high quality and wide range of both the large and targeted trials it offers. Recent changes in its leadership and day-to-day management created an opportunity to re-evaluate how the study start-up cycle time could be reduced without allocating additional staff or financial resources. The project, led by the

NCCCR manager, was strongly supported by the NCCCR and Tufts Medical Center Research Administration leadership.

In health care, cross-functional QI teams often are assembled to diagnose process-based quality problems and develop and test process improvements [6]. Cross-functional teamwork aims to capitalize on the varied knowledge and perspectives of team members, encouraging collaboration that is expected to lead to better problem-solving, more innovative decisions, and greater engagement in implementing the proposed solutions [7]. The process of clinical trial start-up is complex and involves investigators and their study teams, administrative and clinical staff, internal and external Institutional Review Boards (IRB), sponsors, and clinical research organizations, among others. For this CRPI project, engaging all of these stakeholders was considered essential to obtaining an array of perspectives on the clinical trial start-up process and strategies for improving it.

QI methods seek to align teams around a common improvement goal and help diverse groups of stakeholders focus on achieving their collective outcome. Instead of placing blame on individuals for inefficiency, quality improvement theory stresses the importance of examining and addressing systems and processes [8]. From a team-building perspective, this approach creates a safe space for teams to stay motivated and allows members to provide honest feedback about failures that are present in the system. Improvement teams often include a QI expert who provides education and guidance on using QI methods and best practices for designing, implementing and measuring the effectiveness of operational changes. Other team members include individuals knowledgeable about the process being addressed as well as leaders who can be instrumental in motivating and facilitating change. At the core of the team are the individuals who perform the tasks within the process and who would be most impacted by any system changes.

Our cross-functional project team included NCCCR staff as well as representatives with other research roles in the organization and CRPI staff (Table 17.1). The team met bi-weekly for 6 months, rotating in team members as their area of expertise was needed depending on the content being developed each week. For example,

Table 17.1 Team members

Team members
NCCCR Manager[a]
Clinical research coordinators (CRCs)
Institutional review board manager
TMC Grants and contracts manager
NCCCR budget administrator
CRPI Director[a]
CRPI project Manager[a]
CRPI project Coordinator[a]
Research administration staff
Investigational pharmacy representative
NCCCR principal investigators
Research information technology director

[a]Core team member

we engaged the Grants and Contracts Manager to help develop content around executing contracts to ensure our description of and assumptions about the processes were correct. Table 17.1 lists all core team members and additional participants who contributed specialized content.

Understanding the Related Processes and Determining Underlying Causes of Study Start-up Delays

Two of the essential initial steps in the QI process are understanding the related system processes and determining the underlying causes of the problem. Brainstorming sessions and stakeholder interviews were conducted with individuals involved in each step in the study start-up process to ensure that the team had a full understanding of the related processes and reasons for delays. Research coordinators, principal investigators (PIs), and research administrators described the numerous operational challenges they faced in understanding and keeping on top of the study start-up process. IRB, contracting, and budgeting staff explained the common mistakes, delays, and miscommunications they encountered. These themes were then compiled and categorized using a cause-and-effect diagram—a graphical tool for displaying a list of causes associated with a specific effect. (See Fig. 17.1.) The

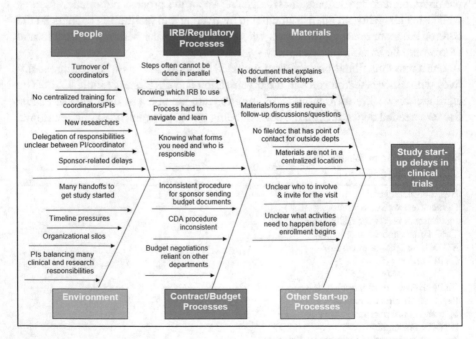

Fig. 17.1 Cause-and-effect diagram displaying the team's consensus of the factors that contribute to study start-up delays

cause-and-effect diagram was reviewed with participants and iteratively revised until participants believed it represented their understanding of the problem.

After consolidating information gathered from our conversations with stakeholders, two central themes emerged: (1) coherent and comprehensive guidance about the start-up process was not available in an accessible format, and (2) institutional knowledge was often lost due to staff turnover. A lack of centralized resources delineating the current process from start to finish led to delays in execution and missed, incomplete, and incorrect actions. The department had standard operating procedures stored in different folders on its shared network drive, but these did not address every aspect of the process and were not organized in a way that facilitated their use. A high rate of research coordinator turnover led to loss of knowledge about established best practices and left research staff struggling to determine how to move the study forward and whom to contact with questions about regulatory, contracting, budgeting, and pharmacy practices.

The CRPI team interviewed research administration staff as well as research coordinators about their knowledge of the tasks and order of the current start-up process and then used this information to draft a composite high level process map. This process map was reviewed by the NCCCR manager and select NCCCR PIs to ensure their agreement with the depiction of the process. This allowed all participants to visualize the current process and achieve a shared knowledge and understanding of each step [8]. In creating the initial map, it became clear that the complexity of the overall process, and varied activities for different types of trials, were important issues. Through repeated revisions of the process map and efforts to seek clarification, the team reached consensus on what the future process should be (See Fig. 17.2). QI tools like process maps are critical for broadly engaged team

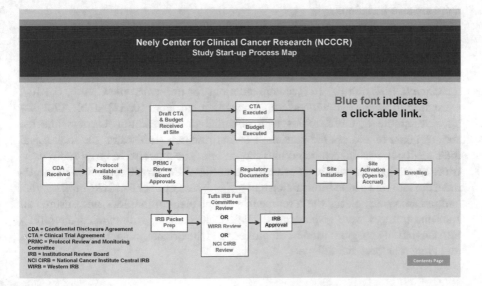

Fig. 17.2 Study start-up process map

science and are effective at reducing confusion, clarifying procedures, and creating buy-in to improve processes that affect multiple stakeholders [9].

Developing and Implementing Changes: The Study Start-Up Toolkit

The process map provided an overview of study start-up, but we also needed a comprehensive set of resources detailing each specific step. The team decided that an extensive toolkit was necessary to address the lack of knowledge about the overall process and the need for uniform policies, procedures, and easily understood guidelines. The process map served as a unifying visual tool to communicate the entire process and link research staff to resources.

Team members gathered relevant documents, examples, and templates to create the toolkit's content. NCCCR staff compiled materials located in disparate locations to a central online file and created hyperlinks within the toolkit to all relevant templates, forms, and guidance documents for easy access. IRB, grants and contracts, pharmacy, and research administration staff contributed detailed descriptions about how to complete study start-up tasks for their areas of responsibility. Each step in the start-up process was described within the toolkit and included background information, detailed instructions, and links to all resource materials. An example of a toolkit page describing steps taken once a protocol is available at the site is depicted in Fig. 17.3. The page provides background on the typical contents of a study protocol, the purpose of a feasibility questionnaire, and tips for study start-up. A description of related process steps and a link to an example feasibility questionnaire are also included.

Once the toolkit was drafted, it was evaluated in a pilot test aimed at assessing potential implementation barriers. This helped ensure that the resource accomplished the intended goals and increased the level of stakeholder engagement and buy-in. Two additional tools, the Consolidated Framework for Implementation Research (CFIR) and Expert Recommendations for Implementing Change (ERIC), were used to assess and address implementation barriers [10, 11]. Table 17.2 displays a sample of CFIR topics with potential implementation barriers and the actions taken to address the barriers. PIs and research staff tested the toolkit and their feedback was incorporated into the design. The exercise led to a more user-friendly version that was responsive to the needs of the target audience. To implement the toolkit we held information and training sessions for NCCCR investigators and research staff, placed the resource in a shared electronic folder, and ensured all staff and trainees were given access. The NCCCR manager integrated the toolkit into the training program for new employees and the orientation of new clinical staff including residents and fellows.

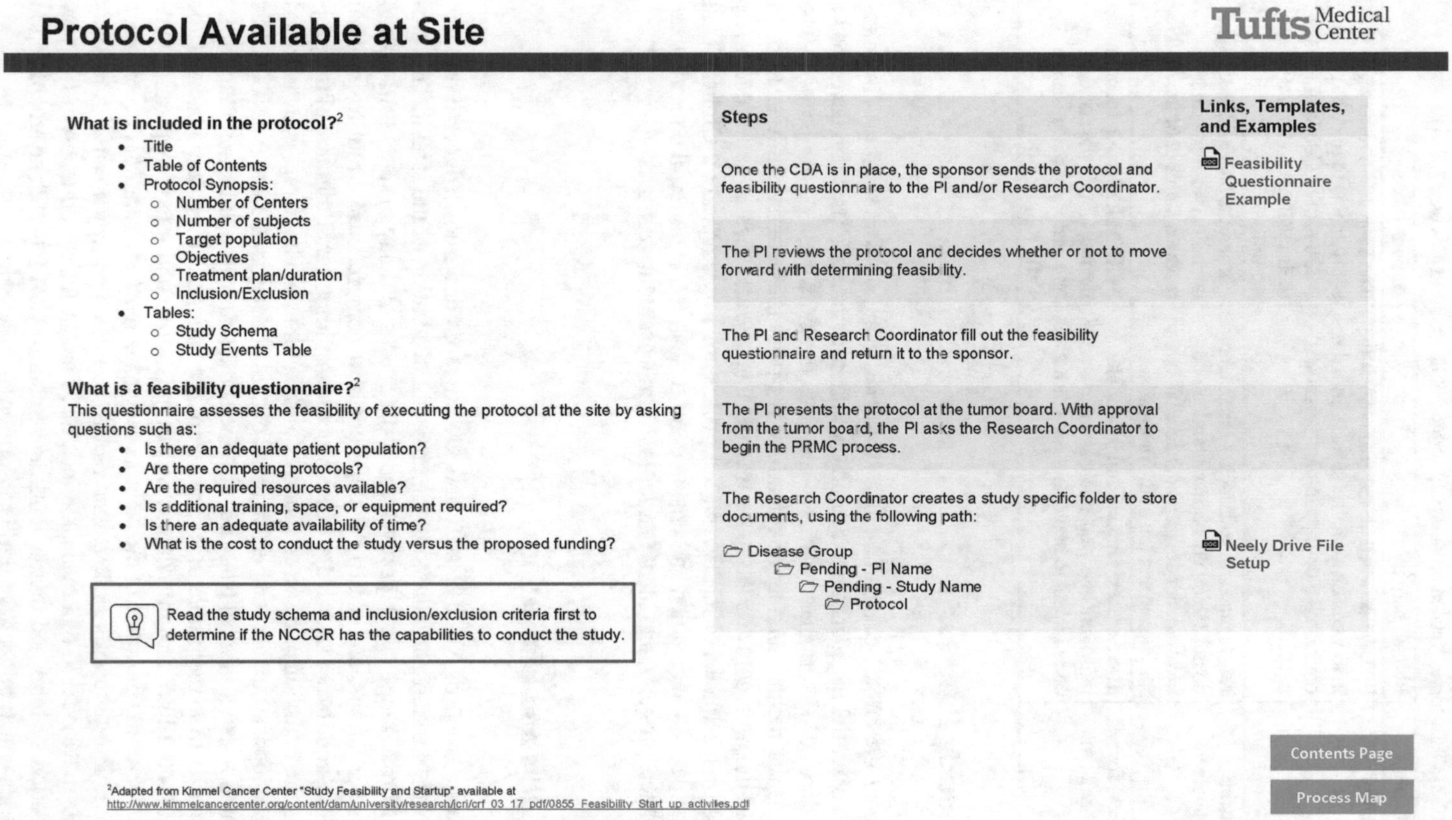

Tufts Medical Center

Protocol Available at Site

What is included in the protocol?[2]

- Title
- Table of Contents
- Protocol Synopsis:
  - Number of Centers
  - Number of subjects
  - Target population
  - Objectives
  - Treatment plan/duration
  - Inclusion/Exclusion
- Tables:
  - Study Schema
  - Study Events Table

What is a feasibility questionnaire?[2]

This questionnaire assesses the feasibility of executing the protocol at the site by asking questions such as:

- Is there an adequate patient population?
- Are there competing protocols?
- Are the required resources available?
- Is additional training, space, or equipment required?
- Is there an adequate availability of time?
- What is the cost to conduct the study versus the proposed funding?

> Read the study schema and inclusion/exclusion criteria first to determine if the NCCCR has the capabilities to conduct the study.

Steps

Once the CDA is in place, the sponsor sends the protocol and feasibility questionnaire to the PI and/or Research Coordinator.

The PI reviews the protocol and decides whether or not to move forward with determining feasibility.

The PI and Research Coordinator fill out the feasibility questionnaire and return it to the sponsor.

The PI presents the protocol at the tumor board. With approval from the tumor board, the PI asks the Research Coordinator to begin the PRMC process.

The Research Coordinator creates a study specific folder to store documents, using the following path:

- Disease Group
  - Pending - PI Name
    - Pending - Study Name
      - Protocol

Links, Templates, and Examples

📄 Feasibility Questionnaire Example

📄 Neely Drive File Setup

Contents Page

Process Map

[2]Adapted from Kimmel Cancer Center "Study Feasibility and Startup" available at
http://www.kimmelcancercenter.org/content/dam/university/research/pdf/crt_03_17_pdf/0855_Feasibility_Start_up_activites.pdf

Fig. 17.3 Toolkit page example

Table 17.2 CFIR topics, related barriers, and implementation strategies used

CFIR topic	Related barrier	Actions taken
Trialability	Stakeholders believe they cannot test the innovation on a smaller scale within the organization or undo implementation if needed.	The team asked research coordinators to pilot-test sections of the toolkit and used their feedback to further refine the tool.
Leadership engagement	Key organizational leaders or managers do not exhibit commitment and are not involved, nor are they held accountable for implementation of the innovation.	PIs and the NCCCR leadership committed to supporting research staff use of the toolkit.
Readiness for implementation	There are few tangible and immediate indicators of organizational readiness and commitment to implement the innovation.	NCCCR leadership incorporated the toolkit into the standard onboarding of new research staff.

Measuring Progress

Assessing the effectiveness of change strategies using outcome and process measures is essential in order to make rapid cycle improvements. The team developed a study start-up performance metric to measure the timeliness of the process. The metric is the median number of calendar days from the date the study team or PI received the protocol from the sponsor to the date the site became active and ready to enroll participants. NCCCR is in the process of implementing a Clinical Trial Management System which will enable them to seamlessly collect the metric data, assess their progress, and identify additional improvement strategies.

Strengths and Limitations

A diverse group of NCCCR staff and investigators and knowledgeable research administrative staff participated in the project and creation of the toolkit. This provided a broad range of perspectives about the causes of delay in study start-up and potential solutions, and led to development of a comprehensive tool to promote efficiency and shared knowledge of the process. An important limitation of the project was the omission of research sponsors and patient stakeholders. Sponsors could have provided a valuable perspective about causes of delay specific to the NCCCR as compared to other clinical trial sites and the sponsor's own operational roadblocks that contribute to the problem. Patients were not engaged at this stage because the project focused primarily on improving administrative and internal operating processes. Including the voice of the patients may have motivated staff to develop even more efficient processes since patient stories can often convey a sense of urgency and may have offered other valuable insights. Finally, the introduction of two new information systems and remote working related to COVID-19 delayed collection of metrics which might have further informed the process.

Next Steps and Lessons Learned

The study start-up toolkit, and the process through which it was developed, were perceived by NCCCR staff and leadership as useful methods to address research roadblocks. Following the implementation of the NCCCR toolkit, other staff in the research community requested the toolkit be adapted for other types of industry-sponsored studies. The CRPI team again used a broad group of organizational stakeholders and expanded implementation activities to include an online training video and access to the toolkit through the organization's intranet. Additional dissemination activities are underway.

The development of the study start-up toolkit revealed how critical it is to:

1. Engage a diverse group stakeholders. Broad stakeholder engagement may delay reaching a consensus and taking action but engaging these participants ensures an innovation addresses their needs.
2. Take time to listen. Change can be slow and difficult but engaging stakeholders in assessing implementation barriers increases the likelihood of a successful implementation.
3. Plan implementation carefully. A good product, tool, or intervention must be tested many times and in many scenarios with various audiences. It takes a few iterations to get it right. Using implementation frameworks can help ensure an innovation gets adopted.
4. Continuously evaluate processes. After a product is developed, it is essential to build in time periods for continuous review to confirm the process is still accurately depicted. As the industry advances and tasks become more automated, processes should also evolve. Make revisions in a timely fashion to inform key stakeholders of any changes.

Just as in health care, QI methods can be used by cross-functional teams of PIs, research staff, and organizational research administrators to plan and execute a continuous flow of improvements in individual studies and the research environment. These improvement teams can leverage the varied knowledge and perspectives of team members, encouraging collaboration that leads to effective problem solving, innovative solutions, and greater engagement in implementing the proposed changes. We suggest that the research community use QI methods and broadly engage stakeholders to tackle the issues that limit the success of translational science.

Acknowledgements   The success of this project would not have been possible without involving a broadly engaged team. The authors wish to acknowledge the contributions of the following individuals:

Neely Center for Clinical Cancer Research - Amanda Campbell; Rachel Buchsbaum, MD; Paul Mathew, MD; Alexandria Ferreira; Jessie Caldwell.

Institutional Review Board Office – Julie Morelli Novak, CIP; Renee Brody.

Grants and Contracts – Nick Corsaro, JD.

Research Administration – Doug Reichgott, MS; Olivia Lovegreen, MBA; Susan Blanchard.
Study Start-up Toolkit Workgroup- Vidya Iyer, MBBS, CCRP; Sara Couture, MPH; Vanessa Palomo.
This work was supported by the NIH CTSA award: UL1TR002544.

References

1. Lamberti MJ, Wilkinson M, Harper B, Morgan C, Getz K (2018) Assessing study start-up practices, performance, and perceptions among sponsors and contract research organizations. Ther Innov Regul Sci 52(5):572–578
2. Tufts Clinical and Translational Science Institute. Research process improvement. Tufts CTSI website. Updated 2021. https://www.tuftsctsi.org/research-services/research-process-improvement/. Accessed 16 Feb 2021
3. Institute of Medicine (2013) The CTSA program at NIH: opportunities for advancing clinical and translational research. The National Academies Press, Washington, DC. https://doi.org/10.17226/18323
4. Patel T, Rainwater J, Trochim WM, Elworth JT, Scholl L, Dave G (2019) Opportunities for strengthening CTSA evaluation [published correction appears in J Clin Transl Sci. 2020 Jan 20;4(1):74]. J Clin Transl Sci 3(2–3):59–64. Published 2019 Jul 26. https://doi.org/10.1017/cts.2019.387
5. McLaughlin CP, Kaluzny AD, Fried B (2006) Defining quality improvement. In: Continuous quality improvement in health care: theory, implementations and applications. John and Bartlett, Sudbury, pp 3–36
6. McLaughlin CP, Kaluzny AD, Fried B (2006) Understanding and improving team effectiveness. In: Continuous quality improvement in health care: theory, implementations and applications. John and Bartlett, Sudbury, pp 154–188
7. Fay D, Borrill C, Amir Z, Haward R, West MA (2006) Getting the most out of multidisciplinary teams: a multi-sample study of team innovation in health care. J Occup Organ Psychol 79(4):553–567
8. Langley GJ (2014) The improvement guide: a practical approach to enhancing organizational performance. Jossey-Bass, San Francisco
9. Quality Improvement Essentials Toolkit: IHI Institute for Healthcare Improvement (2020). http://www.ihi.org/resources/Pages/Tools/Quality-Improvement-Essentials-Toolkit.aspx
10. Constructs (2019) The consolidated framework for implementation research website. https://cfirguide.org/constructs/
11. Powell BJ, Waltz TJ, Chinman MJ, Damschroder LJ, Smith JL, Matthieu MM et al (2015) A refined compilation of implementation strategies: results from the Expert Recommendations for Implementing Change (ERIC) project. Implementation Sci 10:21. https://doi.org/10.1186/s13012-015-0209-1

Chapter 18
Health Literacy and Broadly Engaged Team Science: How One Study Team Used Plain Language Principles to Share Findings with Affected Communities

Sabrina Kurtz-Rossi, Doug Brugge, and Sylvia Baedorf Kassis

Abstract The Community Assessment of Freeway Exposure and Health Study (CAFEH) is a series of participatory research projects aimed at learning about and addressing air pollution from highways and busy roadways. These research projects depend on scientists and community partners working together to document the impact of exposure to near-highway air pollutants and identify actionable solutions. Ultrafine particles (UFPs) are in traffic-related air pollution and are less than a millionth of a meter in diameter. In immigrant communities in and around Boston, CAFEH had identified associations between UFPs and two cardiac risk factors: blood pressure and measures of systemic inflammation, including C-reactive protein (CRP) in peripheral blood. Disseminating study results to affected communities is fundamental to participatory research and engaging community members in identifying workable solutions. However, both the volume and complexity of the findings made it challenging for the study team to communicate them in ways people could understand. In this chapter, we describe how we applied an environmental health literacy framework and plain language principles to develop materials and messages that affected community members could read, understand, and act upon.

This case was original drafted for the Multi-Regional Clinical Trials (MRCT) Center, Health Literacy in Clinical Research case study library https://mrctcenter.org/health-literacy/tools/overview/casestudies/

S. Kurtz-Rossi (✉)
Tufts University School of Medicine, Boston, MA, USA

Tufts Clinical and Translational Science Institute, Boston, MA, USA

D. Brugge
School of Medicine, University of Connecticut, Farmington, CT, USA

S. Baedorf Kassis
Multi-Regional Clinical Trials Center of Brigham and Women's Hospital and Harvard, Boston, MA, USA
e-mail: sabrina.kurtz_rossi@tufts.edu

© The Author(s), under exclusive license to Springer Nature Switzerland AG 2022
D. Lerner et al. (eds.), *Broadly Engaged Team Science in Clinical and Translational Research*, https://doi.org/10.1007/978-3-030-83028-1_18

We also describe challenges, lessons learned, and plans for continued dialogue and program improvement.

Keywords Environmental health literacy · Community assessment of freeway exposure and health study (CAFEH) · Plain language principles · Near-highway air pollutants · Ultrafine particles · Community-based participatory research

The Community Assessment of Freeway Exposure and Health Study (CAFEH) is a series of participatory research projects aimed at learning about and addressing air pollution from highways and busy roadways. These research projects depend on scientists and community partners working together to document the impact of exposure to near highway air pollutants and identify actionable solutions. Ultrafine particles (UFPs) are in traffic-related air pollution and are less than a millionth of a meter in diameter. In immigrant communities in and around Boston, CAFEH had identified associations between UFPs and two cardiac risk factors: blood pressure and measures of systemic inflammation including C-reactive protein (CRP) in peripheral blood [1–4]. Disseminating study results to affected communities is fundamental to participatory research and is increasingly regarded as a necessary element of engaging community members in identifying workable solutions. However, both the volume and complexity of the findings made it challenging for the study team to communicate them in ways people could understand. In addition, many residents were new immigrants who do not speak English as their first language.

In this chapter, we describe our efforts to engage immigrant communities in Boston Chinatown and East Sommerville in identifying and implementing strategies to reduce exposure to near highway UFPs. We highlight the use of an iterative process to develop materials and messages in English, Spanish, Portuguese, and Haitian Creole, which affected community members could read, understand, and act upon.

CAFEH is committed to broadly engaged team science and the full participation of community partners and university-based scientists in all aspects of the research. This includes working together to develop proposals, recruit study participants, collect, analyze and interpret data, report and disseminate findings, and identify and implement solutions. CAFEH research projects are funded primarily by the National Institute for Environmental Health Sciences. Doug Brugge, a public health professor, and Ellin Reisner, head of a community-based advocacy organization, have been Principal Investigators and are committed to exploring the role of environmental health literacy in communicating about UFPs with affected communities.

Environmental Health Literacy

Environmental health literacy as an area of study and practice has been an important part of CAFEH's work. Environmental health literacy prioritizes clear communication between scientists and the community, a common understanding of the problem from an individual and systems level, and critical dialogue about environmental exposure and ways to protect human health [5]. Explaining and understanding the emerging science linking exposure to UFPs and adverse health effects is difficult; collaboratively identifying and implementing ideas and approaches for what to do about it is even more challenging.

Clear communication is needed to create understanding, build trust, and engage community members in collaborative problem-solving. Plain language is a strategic response and a tool in the environmental health literacy toolkit to foster clear communication and transparency in environmental health research.

Plain Language Principles

Clear communication between researchers and the community is a first step to achieving environmental health literacy. Plain language writing and design principles refer to theory-informed techniques that make written materials easy to read [6, 7]. For example, limiting the amount of information, organizing information in manageable chunks, and adding clearly defined headers helps reduce the cognitive load and mental effort for readers (Fig. 18.1).

The CAFEH team applied plain language writing and design principles to communicate what ultrafine particles are and how they may affect human health. We also developed easy-to-read fact sheets describing CAFEH findings. The first iteration of these fact sheets was written in English and translated into Spanish by bilingual study team members. We then conducted focus groups with study participants who reviewed the fact sheets and provided feedback. What we learned from the first two focus groups with Spanish speaking adults (n=16) was that they felt

Plain Language Writing Principles	**Plain Language Design Principles**
• Write in everyday language	• Leave lots of white space on the page
• Define unfamiliar terms	• Increase font size to 12 point or larger
• Use conversational tone	• USE UPPER AND LOWER CASE, NOT ALL CAPS
• Use shorter words and sentences	• *Avoid italic, scripts, fancy fonts*
• Avoid abbreviations and acronyms	• Use **BOLD**, concise headers
• Write in active voice	• Left justify, keep ragged right edge
• Give pro-nun-see-AY-shuns if needed	• Select colors with high contrast

Fig. 18.1 Plain language writing and design principles

overwhelmed by the amount of information in the fact sheets. They found the information confusing, difficult to understand, and lacking in detail about what to do. After revising the fact sheets based on this feedback, we held two more focus groups with the same participants. In these sessions, the participants said they found the information "much easier to read." We learned that larger font size and chunking text improved reading ease, but also realized that there was still more we could do to effectively communicate study results and engage affected communities [8]. As a result, we worked with a health literacy specialist to draft a second series of fact sheets (Fig. 18.2).

We worked with our community partners to translate this content into Spanish, Portuguese, and Haitian Creole, relying on their expertise to ensure the translations were accurate and tailored to the local context (Fig. 18.3). Then, we tested the materials with multilingual, English language learners in partnership with a local adult literacy program.

Health and Literacy Partnerships

Working with adult literacy programs is invaluable for engaging representatives from intended audiences and returning information to study participants. Adult literacy programs can also be strong partners for ensuring information is clearly and appropriately communicated, disseminating research results, and motivating change. These programs are trusted by their students who, in turn, are connected to broad networks that can offer insights to make research more relevant and meaningful.

Since CAFEH is considered educational research (and not human subjects research), our work with the adult literacy program including evaluation was exempt from Institutional Review Board (IRB) review. We worked with a local adult literacy program offering English language classes for immigrants to design a process of gathering formative feedback on the fact sheets for beginner, intermediate, and advanced English language learners. The advanced English language learners sat together to read and discuss the fact sheets in English. English language learners who speak Spanish sat together and reviewed the Spanish translations. Portuguese speakers reviewed the materials in Portuguese and Haitian Creole speakers reviewed the fact sheets in Haitian Creole. Each group of adult learners read the fact sheets on their own and then together discussed a series of questions, including:

- What did you learn by reading the fact sheets?
- What did you learn by looking at pictures on the fact sheets?
- What words or concepts did you find hard to understand?
- What words or concepts do you think people you know might find hard to understand?
- What suggestions do you have for improving the fact sheets?

What Can You Do About Ultrafine Particles (UFPs)?

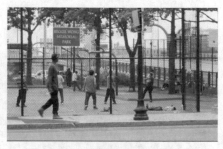

Ultrafine particles (UFPs) are in air near busy roadways. UFPs are also in the air inside homes and buildings near busy roadways.

Here is how you can protect yourself and your family from breathing high levels of ultrafine particles UFPs.

Protect yourself and your family from UFPs near busy roadways.

- **Plan your time <u>outdoors</u> for when UFPs levels are low.**

  Here's when UFPs levels are low outdoors:

  – When there is a breeze in the air

  – When it is warm outside

  – When traffic is light

- **Prevent UFPs from getting <u>indoors</u>.**

  Here's how to keep UFPs levels low indoors:

  – Keep windows closed

  – Use air conditioning or a high-quality air filter

Learn more about ultrafine particles (UFPs) from the Community Assessment of Freeway Exposure and Health Study (CAFEH) https://sites.tufts.edu/cafeh/

Fig. 18.2 An english language fact sheet about UFPs

Adult literacy teachers took notes of group discussions. Because these teachers knew their students' levels of English language proficiency and cultural backgrounds, they were excellent facilitators for us as we improved our communication and cultural understanding. Participants also marked their fact sheets with comments and suggested edits, which were later reviewed by the study team. Feedback was primarily related to word choice and translations, and we revised the fact sheets based accordingly. We also learned that the acronym for ultrafine participles (UFP) did not translate into Portuguese, so we deleted it from that fact sheet.

¿Qué puedes hacer sobre las Partículas Ultrafinas (UFPs)?

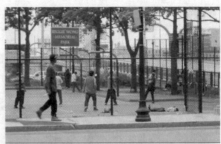

UFPs están en la contaminación del aire cerca de carreteras ocupadas. UFPs también están en el aire dentro de las casas y edificios cerca de carreteras ocupadas.

Así es cómo puedes protegerte y proteger a tu familia de respirar altos niveles de partículas ultrafinas (UFPs).

Protégete y protege a tu familia de UFPs cerca de carreteras ocupadas.

- **Planifique el tiempo afuera para cuando los niveles de UFPs sean bajos.**

  Aquí es cuando los niveles de UFPs son bajos afuera:
  - Cuando hay briza en el aire
  - Cuando está cálido afuera
  - Cuando el tráfico está ligero

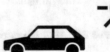

- **Evite que UFPs entren <u>adentro</u>.**
  Así es cómo mantener bajos los niveles de UFPs adentro:
  - Mantén las ventanas cerradas
  - Usa aire acondicionado o un filtro de aire de alta calidad

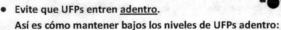

Aprende más sobre partículas ultrafinas (UFPs) del Community Assessment of Freeway Exposure and Health Study (CAFEH) https://sites.tufts.edu/cafeh/

Fig. 18.3 Translation of a fact sheet about UFPs

Successes and Challenges

Paying close attention to the language and culture of the community and collaborating with an adult literacy program helped us engage the community and promote environmental health literacy. Being able to apply plain language writing and design principles to written communications is a critical skill, and not as easy to implement as it may seem. We thought the first set of fact sheets we created were easy to read and understand. However, feedback from study participants indicated that this assumption was incorrect. Even well-intentioned researchers can make inaccurate assumptions about the clarity of their writing for others. To communicate more effectively, we learned to limit the amount of information and use everyday language.

At times, scientists may need to use technical terms to communicate new information and concepts. For example, the subject matter of UFPs includes new terms and concepts that need to be explained. There are many ways to define a word or explain a concept. This is why writing in plain language takes multiple iterations and feedback from the intended audience.

Recommendations for Communicating Complex Research-related Information

Applying a health literacy framework and basic plain language writing and design principles helped us communicate complex research-related information in ways people could understand and use. We also benefited from the input of a health literacy specialist who encouraged us to rethink not only how we tried to explain our research findings and implications, but also how we collaborated with community-based partners. More specifically, the health literacy specialist helped us link the goals of the research team related to disseminating findings with the goals of adult English language learners in terms of learning and practicing relevant language skills. Working with an adult literacy program and directly with English language learners, rather than community activists, was an approach the research team had not tried before. Importantly, translations were also prepared and disseminated for those beginning to learn English and non-English speakers in the broader community.

When communicating with study participants and affected communities, it is critical to engage representatives from your intended audience in developing materials and messages. In our project, we engaged our intended audience in an interactive process of developing easy-to-read materials in multiple language to disseminate research findings related to UFPs in air pollution. Gathering community feedback helps ensure information is accurately and appropriately translated for your intended audience and supports community action.

To learn more visit

- The Community Assessment of Freeway Exposure and Health (CAFEH) https://cafeh.squarespace.com/
- Health Literacy in Clinical Research. Multi-Regional Clinical Trials (MRCT) Center. www.mrctcenter.org/health-literacy

The CAFEH study team continues to look for ways to improve how we communicate study results with affected communities. Future work will include improving our graphic display of information and evaluating the effectiveness of detailed illustrations for communicating the effects of UFPs on human health and what people can do about it. Improving the way we communicate with the public is essential for improving environmental health literacy and health equity overall.

References

1. Walker DI, Lane KJ, Liu K, Uppal K, Patton AP, Durant JL, Jones DP, Brugge D, Pennell KD (2019) Metabolomic assessment of exposure to near-highway ultrafine particles. J Expo Sci Environ Epidemiol 29:469–483
2. Brugge D, Simon MC, Hudda N, Zellmer M, Corlin L, Cleland S, Lu EY, Rivera S, Bryne M, Chung M, Durant JL (2017) Lessons from in-home air filtration intervention trials to reduce urban ultrafine particle number concentrations. Build Environ 126:266–275
3. Fuller CH, O'Neill MS, Sarnat JA, Chang HH, Tucker KL, Brugge D (2018) Short-and medium-term associations of particle number concentration with cardiovascular markers in a Puerto Rican cohort. Environ Res 166:595–601
4. Lane KJ, Levy JI, Scammell MK, Peters JL, Patton AP, Reisner E, Lowe L, Zamore W, Durant J, Brugge D (2016) Association of modeled long-term personal exposure to ultrafine particles with inflammatory and coagulation biomarkers. Environ Int 92-93:173–182
5. Finn S, O'Fallon L (2017) The emergence of environmental health literacy – from its roots to its future potential. Environ Health Perspect 125(4):495–501. https://ehp.niehs.nih.gov/doi/pdf/10.1289/ehp.1409337
6. Kool M, Ruiter RAC, van de Wiel MW, Kok G (2008) The effects of headers in information mapping on search speed and evaluation of a brief health education text. J Inf Sci 34:833–844
7. Gobert R, Lane PC, Croker S, Cheng PC, Jones G, Oliver I, Pine JM (2001) Chunking mechanisms in human learning. Trends Cogn Sci 5(6):236–243
8. Brugge D, Tracy M, Thayer K, Thayer A, Dayer B, Figueroa N, Kurtz-Rossi S (2018) The role of environmental health literacy when developing traffic pollution fact sheets for Puerto Rican adults. Environ Justice 11:40–46. https://www.ncbi.nlm.nih.gov/pmc/articles/PMC5830854/

Chapter 19
Utilizing Patient Navigators to Promote Equitable and Accountable Research

Mingqian Lin, Douglas Hackenyos, Fengqing Wang, Nicole Savidge, Angela Wimmer, Antonia Maloney, Susan Mohebbi, Michele Guard, and Susan K. Parsons

Abstract Over the past decade, studies have shown that patient navigators (PNs) are effective at helping clinical care teams address heath care barriers and improve health outcomes through a patient-centered approach; however, there has been far less consideration of how PNs could facilitate or be involved in research. In this chapter, we present examples illustrating PN's wide spectrum of roles and capabilities in clinical care and explain how these skills could further enrich research teams, particular those aimed at clinical, health services, systems science, and community-based research. PNs can bring patient experiences into research discussions, helping inform topics of investigative interest, study design, and methodology so that they are more reflective and considerate of needs and challenges faced by patients. The inclusion of PNs in research teams could also facilitate broader engagement of stakeholders, particularly populations that are underrepresented in research.

Keywords Patient navigator · Patient navigation · Community-based research

The COVID-19 pandemic in the United States has increased the visibility of health and health care inequities in our nation and has further underscored the importance of conducting health disparity research to improve health outcomes particularly for underserved populations. The term "health disparities" specifically refers to differences in health and health outcomes that disproportionately affect socially and economically disadvantaged populations. Because some health disparities are

M. Lin (✉) ·
Tufts Medical Center, Boston, MA, USA

Medical College of Wisconsin, Milwaukee, WI, USA

D. Hackenyos · F. Wang · N. Savidge · A. Maloney · S. Mohebbi · M. Guard
S. K. Parsons
Tufts Medical Center, Boston, MA, USA

A. Wimmer
University of Arkansas for Medical Sciences, Little Rock, AR, USA

© The Author(s), under exclusive license to Springer Nature
Switzerland AG 2022
D. Lerner et al. (eds.), *Broadly Engaged Team Science in Clinical and Translational Research*, https://doi.org/10.1007/978-3-030-83028-1_19

preventable, as they are largely due to inequality in terms of access, resources, and/ or health beliefs, research can play a large part in addressing this issue [1].

Over the past decade, patient navigation is increasingly implemented in patient care settings to address barriers to health care and improve health outcomes through a patient-centered approach. In 1990, Dr. Harold P. Freeman, a Black surgeon working in the Harlem neighborhood of New York City, noticed that his patients of color were presenting with more advanced colorectal cancer than white patients. He established patient navigation to improve colorectal screening with the goal of reducing cancer disparities. Typically, patient navigators (PNs) are lay individuals or professionals from a variety of disciplinary backgrounds, and while not all may hold a clinical license (in contrast to nurse navigators or social workers, for example), various certificate programs offer more formal training. Patient navigation programs now exist nationwide and provide services across the cancer care continuum: from screening to diagnosis, treatment, survivorship, and/or end of life [2]. In 2012, the American College of Surgeons' Commission on Cancer made the process of identifying health disparities and reducing barriers to care, such as by providing PNs, an accreditation requirement for cancer centers [3]. Given the prevailing need for more comprehensive support in an increasingly complex health care system, patient navigation programs have also been implemented for the management of other diseases, such as cardiovascular disease and diabetes [4, 5].

PNs are important members within a multidisciplinary clinical care team and perform a variety of roles. The PN's role is to assist patients and their caregivers according to their needs, which may include addressing insurance coverage and financial issues; accompanying patients to visits; finding food and transportation; making and coordinating appointments; enhancing patient education; improving patient-provider communication; and bringing awareness of cultural or religious concerns to health care providers [6].

A number of studies have highlighted the potential benefits of utilizing PNs within different disease groups and health care settings. In oncology, the introduction of patient navigation has resulted in better screening rates and follow-up, reduced time to diagnosis, higher patient satisfaction, and improved communication and delivery of culturally sensitive care between health providers, patients, and caregivers [7–10]. Among patients with diabetes, one study found a reduction in appointment no-show rates among uninsured patients, while another study showed improved glycemic control in patients who were assigned PNs [11, 12]. Patients diagnosed with HIV who had support from PNs were also found to have better viral load suppression compared to those without PNs, particularly when they had more frequent communication with their care providers [13].

Underrepresented minorities, low-income and/or uninsured individuals, and individuals with limited English proficiency disproportionately experience worse cancer outcomes and additional barriers to care [14–16]. Because Tufts Medical Center is located in Chinatown in Boston, MA, many of its patients are persons of Chinese origin. From 2011 to 2014, we conducted formative research leading to the establishment of a patient navigation program in the Cancer Center at Tufts Medical Center dedicated to improving the quality of care for patients of lower socioeconomic status and/or of Chinese origin. PNs at Tufts Medical Center work as part of the cancer care team to support patients throughout the expansive trajectory of cancer care: from diagnosis through treatment and into survivorship or end-of-life care. To adequately cover the cancer care spectrum, PNs provide linguistically- and culturally-congruent care as well as support that is longitudinal and tailored to each patient. While the PNs help patients navigate through their challenges, they are also a continual presence, often accompanying patients to their appointments and checking in with them between visits. In these ways they have helped to expand the capacity of the cancer care team to support a patient population with complex, diverse needs.

The majority of patients served by the patient navigation program at Tufts Medical Center also have limited to no English-speaking ability, have low health literacy and educational attainment, and have low income or receive public health insurance. To specifically address the language needs of Chinese patients, we have hired bilingual PNs who are fluent in multiple Chinese dialects. The bilingual PNs have facilitated communications by being able to speak directly with patients, bringing any concerns or questions to the clinical team's attention, and communicating information from the cancer care team to the patients and their caregivers in a timely way. While they do not replace medical interpreters, PNs develop familiarity with their patients' histories and can add context to communicated information using language that is culturally sensitive and appropriate.

In addition, PNs also serve as cultural bridges, bringing awareness of various cultural preferences, traditions, and behaviors to the cancer care team. For example, PNs have cautioned health care providers about the social stigma of cancer when recommending support groups to Chinese patients. During one mediated conversation between a patient and her oncologist, who was initially concerned about the patient's use of a Chinese herbal medicine, the PN helped clarify that the herb was an ingredient used in a common Chinese traditional soup. In another example, a PN was able to advocate for a patient who wanted to start her chemotherapy after the Lunar New Year, a time that is widely regarded as auspicious in Chinese culture. Ultimately, the patient was able to reach a compromise with her cancer care team while enhancing her adherence to therapy.

Integrating Patient Navigators into Research Teams

While PNs have become increasingly important to patient care teams and as a topic of research, so far there appears to be less consideration of how they could facilitate or be involved in research teams. In the following sections, we will expand upon the roles and capabilities of PNs at Tufts Medical Center Cancer Center and describe how these same skills could augment research and research teams.

Patient Navigators Expand Research Participation

PNs are liaisons across the health care provider and layperson clinical and cultural divides, possessing a unique skill set and knowledge base that synthesizes different perspectives and information. Their unique background and their close relationships with patients, caregivers, and providers can similarly help bridge the divide between academia and the public. PNs can help inform research study and program development by obtaining input and perspectives from patients and caregivers so that research questions and intervention goals address relevant issues. For example, during the development of the patient navigation program at Tufts Medical Center Cancer Center, PNs developed and conducted a series of qualitative interviews to learn about our patients' experiences of their cancer care. The results of these interviews helped guide the direction and services of our navigation program to address actual patient needs. Additionally, PNs can assist in study recruitment and enrollment, not only by overcoming language barriers, but also by cultivating better understanding of research and a greater sense of trust, which may be especially important for many underserved populations. Given their familiarity with the clinical space and processes, and their rapport with providers, PNs can also help with the implementation of studies. They can assist in participant follow-up, checking in for any questions and concerns and communicating them to the research team. They can enable or enhance dissemination of knowledge gained from research to participants and the communities they represent, bridging gaps in communication between the community and research teams.

Patient Navigators Enhance the Ability of Research Teams to Address Diverse Issues

Along with their high level of commitment to supporting comprehensive care for patients, PNs have developed a mindset that leads them to interact with patients and providers holistically. The capacity for PNs to address many different needs, their direct exposure to a range of potential barriers for patients, and their expertise across several areas, including health systems, health care delivery, health education, and clinical trials can add diversity to research teams and research topics.

For example, the PNs at Tufts Medical Center frequently help patients overcome financial, logistical, and insurance barriers, and they are often called upon to solve challenges related to transportation and food access, billing issues, and medical leave and unemployment assistance. PNs have also worked with patients in obtaining insurance coverage (e.g., applying for Medicaid or MassHealth) or browsing through different insurance products. They have helped patients navigate through different and fragmented health systems and organizations (i.e., hospitals, insurance companies, pharmacies, and specialty pharmacies) so that these systems, lines of communications, and information are consolidated and streamlined. Given the high cost of cancer care, the addition of new logistical burdens associated with treatment and follow-up, and the convoluted insurance system in the United States, PNs have become valuable resources for our patients. Their knowledge of the health system and the patient experience of health systems barriers adds useful insight to research topics and interventions dedicated to these issues.

In addition, PNs often have experience improving the delivery and quality of care. This experience can guide research teams to develop studies aimed at enhancing cancer care delivery, an emerging research priority within cancer centers. The introduction of PNs at Tufts Medical Center Cancer Center has led to several efforts to enhance supports and services for the providers, patients, and caregivers. First, the PNs have become extensions to the clinicians and helped expand their capacity to care for their patients. Clinicians have regularly utilized the navigators to coordinate appointments (e.g., routine follow-up, infusion treatments, diagnostic and surveillance testing) to help reduce delays and promote adherence to care. PNs have also frequently checked in with patients in between their visits to review symptoms and treatment side effects and relay them promptly to the cancer care team for timely resolution. PNs have worked with social workers and palliative care providers to facilitate discussions on palliative and end-of-life care with Chinese patients, while raising awareness of the need for more culturally appropriate resources and services for these sensitive topics. Additionally, pharmacists have worked extensively with the PNs to resolve issues with refills and obtaining prescriptions and medications. The inclusion of PNs in the delivery of care has identified limitations and barriers to care and introduced potential solutions to address them. The insights of PNs in care delivery can serve as valuable knowledge that can directly be applied in research. Furthermore, their inclusion in clinical care teams allows them to offer care experiences to research teams from the perspectives of patients and providers.

PNs at Tufts Medical Center have also been utilized in patient education and clinical trials and can assist research teams to improve patient awareness and education, participant recruitment, and trial implementation. Oncologists and nurses have frequently invited PNs to participate in chemotherapy teaching to ensure that patients better understand the information. The PNs help present information in a way that is better understood (i.e., eliminating medical jargon), which we found to be especially helpful for patients with low health literacy or education attainment. In 2018, a study initiative was implemented at Tufts Medical Center Cancer Center to enhance understanding, adherence, and support for patients newly starting on oral anti-cancer medications through formalized teaching and follow-up sessions with Tufts Medical Center Cancer Center's oncology specialty pharmacist and PNs. While the PNs were a feature of the intervention, they were also enlisted in the research team. They were able to offer insights about medication-related issues, explaining what the patients' challenges were and how they could be addressed in the study's goals and methodology. They also aided in the development of the study's educational materials (information sheets about the oral anti-cancer medications) by tailoring them to our patient population to optimize their understanding.

PNs at Tufts Medical Center have also elevated awareness and understanding of cancer treatment clinical trials, which continue to evoke caution and apprehension particularly among many underserved and ethnic minority populations [17]. In one case, a patient was able to overcome her reluctance about enrolling in an NCI-sponsored clinical trial as a result of PN and social worker interventions. Specifically, the PN's empathy and understanding of the cultural stigma around cancer helped her to educate the patient about the trial and assuage her fears. The PN also facilitated the involvement of the social worker to focus on the patient's social and personal concerns. This partnership better equipped the cancer care team to address the complex and multifaceted barriers for the patient to enroll in the trial and obtain treatment [18].

Preparing and Supporting Patient Navigators in Research

The prior examples illustrate the PN's wide spectrum of roles and capabilities in clinical care, while also showcasing skills that can further enrich research teams. The broad and diverse knowledge and experiences that PNs possess, some of which are encapsulated by the examples we presented, portray the versatility of PNs to be involved in different types of research (e.g., clinical, health services, systems science, community-based research). They also bring patient experiences into research discussions, which can help inform topics of investigative interest, study design, and methodology so that they are more reflective and considerate of existing barriers and challenges faced by patients.

The ways in which PNs are integrated into research teams and what roles they play will need to be further explored. Current training programs primarily emphasize preparing potential PNs to function in health care and clinical settings [6]. Therefore, PNs may have less preparation and experience in academic research. As PNs become a more common presence across health care settings and in multidisciplinary teams, existing training programs may consider supplementing their curricula with information about fundamental research processes, including different types of studies and study sponsors. The addition of PNs to research teams will likely require new sources of fiscal support or expansion of current research funding mechanisms to ensure adequate training, supervision, and support.

To reflect the expanding health needs of an increasingly diverse population, we must continue to consider ways of conducting research that engage individuals in effective and meaningful ways. The potential for health research to transform and improve the lives of individuals facing health inequities remains a goal. PNs traditionally have not been incorporated into research teams but can be utilized to facilitate broader engagement of stakeholders through their unique training, particularly for populations that are underrepresented in research. Through the patient-centeredness of their work, PNs can hold research teams more accountable and drive research towards addressing issues that are impactful. Team diversity not only emphasizes multidisciplinary collaboration, but also highlights the importance of team equity. It is crucial that these broader perspectives and backgrounds not only be included, but that each individual holds equal weight in the conversation. By endorsing equity in contributions from all members, research teams become more accountable and more effective at improving outcomes.

References

1. CDC (2008) Community Health and Program Services (CHAPS): health disparities among racial/ethnic populations. U.S. Department of Health and Human Services, Atlanta
2. Freeman HP, Rodriguez RL (2011) History and principles of patient navigation. Cancer 117(15 Suppl):3539–3542. https://doi.org/10.1002/cncr.26262
3. Cancer Program Standards 2012: Ensuring Patient-Centered Care (2012) Commission on cancer. 2012 American College of Surgeons, Chicago
4. Scott LB, Gravely S, Sexton TR, Brzostek S, Brown DL (2013) Examining the effect of a patient navigation intervention on outpatient cardiac rehabilitation awareness and enrollment. J Cardiopulm Rehabil Prev 33(5):281–291. https://doi.org/10.1097/HCR.0b013e3182972dd6
5. English TM, Masom D, Whitman MV (2018) The impact of patient navigation on diabetes. J Healthc Manag 63(3):e32–e41. https://doi.org/10.1097/JHM-D-16-00033
6. Willis A, Hoffler E, Villalobos A, Pratt-Chapman M (2016) Advancing the field of cancer patient navigation: a toolkit for comprehensive cancer control professionals. The George Washington University Cancer Institute, Washington, DC
7. Reuland DS, Brenner AT, Hoffman R, McWilliams A, Rhyne RL, Getrich C, Tapp H, Weaver MA, Callan D, Cubillos L, Urquieta de Hernandez B, Pignone MP (2017) Effect of combined patient decision aid and patient navigation vs usual care for colorectal cancer screening in a vulnerable patient population: a randomized clinical trial. JAMA Intern Med 177(7):967–974. https://doi.org/10.1001/jamainternmed.2017.1294
8. Ferrante JM, Chen PH, Kim S (2008) The effect of patient navigation on time to diagnosis, anxiety, and satisfaction in urban minority women with abnormal mammograms: a randomized controlled trial. J Urban Health 85(1):114–124. https://doi.org/10.1007/s11524-007-9228-9
9. Jean-Pierre P, Cheng Y, Wells KJ, Freund KM, Snyder FR, Fiscella K, Holden AE, Paskett ED, Dudley DJ, Simon MA, Valverde PA (2016) Satisfaction with cancer care among underserved racial-ethnic minorities and lower-income patients receiving patient navigation. Cancer 122(7):1060–1067. https://doi.org/10.1002/cncr.29902
10. Phillips S, Phillips S, Villalobos AVK, Villalobos AVK, Crawbuck GSN, Crawbuck GSN, Pratt-Chapman ML, Pratt-Chapman ML (2019) In their own words: patient navigator roles in culturally sensitive cancer care. Support Care Cancer 27(5):1655–1662. https://doi.org/10.1007/s00520-018-4407-7
11. Weaver KR, Talley M, Mullins M, Selleck C (2019) Evaluating patient navigation to improve first appointment no-show rates in uninsured patients with diabetes. J Community Health Nurs 36(1):11–18. https://doi.org/10.1080/07370016.2018.1555315
12. Horny M, Glover W, Gupte G, Saraswat A, Vimalananda V, Rosenzweig J (2017) Patient navigation to improve diabetes outpatient care at a safety-net hospital: a retrospective cohort study. BMC Health Serv Res 17(1):759. https://doi.org/10.1186/s12913-017-2700-7
13. Stitzer M, Matheson T, Cunningham C, Sorensen JL, Feaster DJ, Gooden L, Hammond AS, Fitzsimons H, Metsch LR (2017) Enhancing patient navigation to improve intervention session attendance and viral load suppression of persons with HIV and substance use: a secondary post hoc analysis of the Project HOPE study. Addict Sci Clin Pract 12(1):16. https://doi.org/10.1186/s13722-017-0081-1
14. Siegel RL, Miller KD, Jemal A (2020) Cancer statistics, 2020. CA Cancer J Clin 70(1):7–30. https://doi.org/10.3322/caac.21590
15. Genoff MC, Zaballa A, Gany F, Gonzalez J, Ramirez J, Jewell ST, Diamond LC (2016) Navigating language barriers: a systematic review of patient navigators' impact on cancer

screening for limited English proficient patients. J Gen Intern Med 31(4):426–434. https://doi.org/10.1007/s11606-015-3572-3

16. Timmins CL (2002) The impact of language barriers on the health care of Latinos in the United States: a review of the literature and guidelines for practice. J Midwifery Womens Health 47(2):80–96. https://doi.org/10.1016/s1526-9523(02)00218-0

17. Paterniti DA, Chen MS, Beckett LA, Chiechi C, Horan NM, Turrell C, Darr J, Gonzalez J, Davis S, Lara PN (2005) Understanding Asian American awareness of and experience with cancer clinical trials (CCTs): a mixed methods approach. J Clin Oncol 23(16_suppl):6052. https://doi.org/10.1200/jco.2005.23.16_suppl.6052

18. Parsons SK, Fineberg IC, Lin M, Singer M, Tang M, Erban JK (2016) Promoting high-quality cancer care and equity through disciplinary diversity in team composition. J Oncol Pract 12(11):1141–1147. https://doi.org/10.1200/JOP.2016.013920

Chapter 20
Asian American Research in the Post-Atlanta Era: Driving Community-Engaged Research That Is More Meaningful, Responsive, and Actionable for Local Communities

Carolyn Leung Rubin, Ben Hires, Dawn Sauma, and Yoyo Yau

Abstract Since its founding in 2011, Addressing Disparities in Asian Populations through Translational Research (ADAPT), a collaboration between Tufts Medical Center, Tufts University, and Boston Chinatown community partners, has aimed to raise awareness of Asian health disparities and facilitate community-engaged research that addresses the health of Asian Americans "We make the path by walking it"; building an academic community partnership with Boston Chinatown. Prog Community Health Partnersh 8(3):353–363. https://doi.org/10.1353/cpr.2014.0046). This chapter will briefly review the significant challenges facing Asian American health research, how we have encountered those challenges in our work at ADAPT, and ways that we have learned to overcome barriers and focus on priorities identified by the community we serve.

Keywords Disparities in Asian populations · Asian health disparities · Data equity · ADAPT

Since its founding in 2011 by a group of Chinatown partners, Asian clinicians, and Tufts researchers, Addressing Disparities in Asian Populations through Translational

C. L. Rubin (✉)
Tufts University School of Medicine, Boston, MA, USA

B. Hires · Y. Yau
Boston Chinatown Neighborhood Center, Boston, MA, USA

D. Sauma
Asian Task Force Against Domestic Violence, Boston, MA, USA
e-mail: Carolyn.Rubin@tufts.edu

© The Author(s), under exclusive license to Springer Nature Switzerland AG 2022
D. Lerner et al. (eds.), *Broadly Engaged Team Science in Clinical and Translational Research*, https://doi.org/10.1007/978-3-030-83028-1_20

Research (ADAPT) has worked to build academic-community partnerships to support research on Asian health equity issues, as defined by the community and using community-engaged research approaches [1]. ADAPT partners include Tufts Medical Center, Tufts University, and various Boston Chinatown community partners, such as the Asian Task Force Against Domestic Violence, Asian Women for Health, Action for Boston Community Development/Chinese Church Head Start, Asian Community Development Corporation, Boston Chinatown Neighborhood Center, and the Greater Boston Chinese Golden Age Center. This chapter will briefly review the evolution of ADAPT, the significant organizational challenges ADAPT has encountered while conducting local Asian American health research, and what we have learned about overcoming these challenges and focusing on priorities identified by the community we care about and are responsible to.

Challenges Facing Asian American Health Research: Lack of Understanding of Community, Racism, and Data Equity

Building trust between academic institutions and underserved communities is a complex and challenging undertaking. Underserved communities are wary of researchers who want to use them for their benefit without really giving back to the community in meaningful ways. As a result of certain historical events, building trust was a particular challenge for ADAPT. In the 1950s, a major highway was constructed through Boston Chinatown, literally dividing it in half. Then, in the 1970s and 1980s the City of Boston, took almost one-third of the land of Chinatown by eminent domain to facilitate the expansion of Tufts University's medical campus, razing buildings, displacing families, and destroying key social networks because residents' homes were seen disparagingly as "tenements." Some claim that the long-term impacts of these institutional actions are still felt today as the residents of Chinatown continue to grapple with the need for affordable housing, the impact of highway pollution, and everyday racism [2].

Asian American advocates often talk about themselves as the invisible, misunderstood, and forgotten minority. Few know that many Chinese immigrants initially came to this country as laborers from a particular province in China. They were actively recruited to replace outlawed slave labor and were brought here to help build the transcontinental railroad, often being given the most dangerous jobs [3]. Locally, Tufts faculty, students, and staff mention that they walk around the neighborhood but have no knowledge of its history, challenges, and ongoing fight to maintain its resiliency. As recently as 1993, residents of Chinatown had to fight against Tufts Medical Center's plans to turn a portion of their neighborhood into a parking lot. The residents prevailed and a mixed-use building of market rate and affordable housing was developed, including permanent space for critical non-profit organizations serving the neighborhood.

ADAPT is doing its work as a research entity in the context of and because of this troubled history of medical research and underserved communities in Boston, which includes a collective historical amnesia about and disregard for the neighborhood's history among Tufts and other institutions. Additionally, ADAPT's work is necessitated by the implicit bias and racism created by invisibility, misrepresentations, and lack of understanding of the Asian community, which plays out in research and the institutions responsible for producing relevant data. The model minority thesis developed by sociologist William Patterson was popularized in his 1966 *New York Times* and the 1987 *TIME Magazine* article about "the Whiz Kids," solidifying in the American consciousness that Asians should be heralded as an immigrant group who has "made it" in America [4, 5]. While many Asian American academics have written about and provided empirical data to refute the model minority thesis, it is at the basis of racism that overshadows the national Asian American community and hurts, in particular, working-class Asian immigrant communities like Chinatown. Arguably, this framing of the Asian American success story was a strategic move to create tension among other Black, Indigenous, and other communities of color (BIPOC) so they would fight over scarce resources, divide communities, and detract from the real fight against systemic racism.

Data have been used against the Asian American community in other ways as well. At the national level, the Asian American community is a heterogeneous group that differs by socio-economic status, language, immigration status, and education level. When data about these diverse Asian American sub-groups are lumped together, key life outcomes such as education, income, and health do not always indicate disparities or inequities. However, when the data are disaggregated into subgroups, then a bi-modal distribution of characteristics in terms of education, income, and health are evident. For example, in a gentrified neighborhood like Boston Chinatown, there is a difference between the income of Chinese who live in the area and non-Chinese residents who live in nearby high-end luxury buildings. In addition, between 2000 and 2018 median area income for Chinese residents went down from $19,171 to $17,997 while area median income for White residents rose from $42,710 to $113,678 [6]. Examples like this illustrate that for data to be useful to the community, it must also be contextualized.

Community partners in neighborhoods like Chinatown and Dorchester (which is heavily Vietnamese) worry that data that is not locally driven masks the challenges that their working-class immigrant constituencies face, many of whom work in industries like restaurants and nail salons and have lost their jobs but may not seek unemployment claims. Without a recognition of the limitations of this data, this type of data actually hurts the community because it reinforces the model minority myth and makes it difficult for community members to make their case with philanthropic organizations and government funders, who are already working from an unexamined place of implicit bias towards Asians and who provide funding for community services.

When ADAPT started in 2011, community partners immediately alerted us to the fact that the Boston Public Health Commission does not consider Chinatown its own neighborhood and so, Chinatown health data is combined with data from one of its abutting neighborhoods, the South End. However, Chinatown and the South End differ from each other by race and class. Chinatown community agencies have pointed to this treatment of data as hampering its ability to secure funding to address community needs. One of the community agencies, the Boston Chinatown Neighborhood Center (BCNC), approached ADAPT with this problem. One of the ADAPT academics took this on as a challenge to get public health surveillance data about the Chinatown community. She submitted a grant to the Tufts Clinical and Translational Science Institute (CTSI) Pilot Awards Program and the proposal was rejected. One of the cited reasons was that the project was not "innovative" and did not have a "clear hypothesis." Subsequently, this researcher was able to secure a $50,000 grant from Tufts Collaborates, an internal funding mechanism of the Tufts University Office of Vice-Provost for Research, to work with BCNC to conduct a population-based, representative survey using questions from the Behavioral Risk Factor Surveillance System Survey, which is a tool that the Boston Public Health Commission uses. This funding source understood the need for local, community-specific data.

Building Trust Between Academics and Community Partners

Learning how to build and sustain community-academic trust has been foundational to the work of ADAPT. When Tufts had the opportunity to apply for Center of Excellence grants from the National Institute of Minority Health Disparities within the National Institutes of Health (NIH), the intensive grant period tested this trust. During the first round, ADAPT received a high score and we were lauded for our strong authentic community engagement. Even so, the trust we had built was tested because there was a difference between what community partners wanted to focus on—mental health—and what Tufts researchers had expertise in, namely cancer and diabetes. Community partners understand the nature of grantsmanship and were willing to take the chance on a new topic because they felt that this grant could help leverage other grants more aligned with the community. One community partner said in confidence, "What's worse, not getting the grant or getting the grant and us spending five years implementing something that we, as the community, are not as excited about?" Other community partners expressed frustration because they were physically at the table during research discussion, yet they did not always find the discussions accessible. This underscores the kind of compromises community partners have made to build relationships with large academic institutions from which they are trying to leverage funds to support community needs. After the process was over, community partners appreciated how hard the academics worked to write the grant; however, they also felt the need to meet privately to discuss concerns about the process and partnership. Because the academics listened, the relationship was strengthened. In the end, though, despite the score, the NIH Council did not award ADAPT the grant.

We did have a second opportunity to write an NIH Center of Excellence grant. Unlike the previous time, however, despite reviewer comments about the strength of community engagement, the application did not get a score, which meant that it had no chance of being considered for funding. A few of the weaknesses cited included, (1) "Minimal justification for focusing exclusively on Chinese populations, other than long-standing relationships between researchers and this community" and (2) "Focus on persons of Chinese descent living in Boston Chinatown limits generalizability and broader applicability."

While it is true that there are other Asian ethnic groups living in the Boston area, it is troubling to think that Chinatown is too small a geographic area because it lacks the potential for generalizability. Both of the critiques illustrate a lack of understanding of the heterogeneity of the Asian American community, our different histories, challenges, and assets. Given the heterogeneity of any racial group, it also brings into question whether generalizability should always be the goal of research or whether it is also important to understand the unique needs of small yet significant populations. It is difficult to imagine that work on a neighborhood like Boston Chinatown—a vibrant neighborhood with a unique history and specific health issues—should not be studied because of its small numbers and therefore lack of generalizability. Community history and context matters. The first comment also lacked an understanding of authentic community engagement. Long-standing relationships are a strength that should be honored. While reviewers are not to be expected to understand the history, community, and character of every different community, it does beg the question of what reviewers believe is the purpose of community engagement. Is community engagement window dressing or stamp of approval for what researchers want, what the limited literature base says (with the peer review process as a gatekeeper), or do they actually honor and respect community priorities and self determination? If community stakeholders say, "this is what is best for our community" is that truly honored? Or is community engagement still filtered through what a researcher thinks should happen, and is local, community expertise still not as valued an academic expertise, which is an issue of power? The knowledge, skills, and expertise that comes from lived experience and practice-based experience should be seen, compensated, and respected on an equal footing. For example, why isn't cultural and linguistic expertise seen and compensated as a specialization, the way medical specialties are? Skills sets and expertise of academics and community partners need to be seen as equally important, valued, and compensated so that the work can be complementary and synergistic, fueled by true power sharing and honest dialogue.

ADAPT's Evolution: Focus on Community-identified Priorities and Moving Research to Practice

Misalignment between community priorities and academic expertise continued to challenge ADAPT, particularly for NIH grants, which require demonstrated expertise in a particular area. Because of these challenges, our community engagement process evolved. We have focused on giving our partners the space to define what health looks like and means for our Chinatown community. Moving from population health to a place-based perspective, ADAPT has concentrated on health priorities as defined by our community partners. These are health projects, defined outside the biomedical definition of health that address urgent and invisible needs expressed by community, particularly in the era of rapid displacement in Chinatown. Over the last few years, two community partners asked to collaborate with ADAPT on housing, art and health, and problem gambling. While these are not "typical" health issues, they fundamentally contribute to upstream approaches to health and overall quality of life.

The success of two of these community-identified research projects has allowed us to see the potential to move from research to practice. Asian CARES, a regional coalition of services providers that span Chinatown, Dorchester, and Lowell has already attracted the attention of community stakeholders, residents, and policymakers (e.g., the Chinatown City Council and the Department of Public Health) who are interested in gathering data that support the need for increased funding for treatment and prevention services in the Asian community. The Asian CARES Coalition is emerging as the leading voice, convener, and advocacy group addressing problem gambling in the region. The Pao Arts Center is collaborating with the University of Florida, Arts and Health, which has been funded by the National Endowment for the Arts to use large-scale epidemiological data to make the case for arts as a form of medicine. This working group is developing a policy and advocacy platform to not just highlight the importance of arts on health but to find ways for it to be integrated into healthcare and the healing modalities offered to patients. In addition, the Health and Housing project, funded by Tufts Collaborates, gave the Asian Community Development Corporation the opportunity to look at the relationship between health and housing. The challenge, however, with many of these community-based grants is that they do not adequately fund the researcher or the community partner to truly bring the project through to translation in the community.

These research projects embody the spirit of ADAPT and the commitment of all partners. They focus on health concerns, as defined by the community. They are co-led and co-constructed with the community. Academics in ADAPT take on these projects even if they are not formally trained in the content areas of expertise. These projects show that if the community partner brings the context expertise, then academic researchers can productively collaborate if they know how to listen, respect, and be responsive to community needs. One of the challenges for academic researchers is that those who rely on NIH grants are expected to build content expertise in one area, which can be at odds with community needs, which are constantly changing and shifting.

We are proud of the work ADAPT has done with our limited resources. We have a Director who devotes 15% of her time to ADAPT and other Stakeholder and Community Engagement work, a part-time Program Manager, and an Asian Health Equity fellow funded by the Department of Public Health and Community Medicine, whose faculty have been the backbone of ADAPT. Tufts CTSI has provided grant writing support to community-led research projects and their professional development team works with ADAPT to plan our annual Asian Health Symposium, which attracts close to 100 people. Our symposium is not a typical academic conference. Instead, we reach out to community leaders, residents, students, clinicians, City and State officials, and researchers. Our most recent Asian Health Symposium adopted the model of having practitioners as discussants, not to play the typical role of critiquing the research, but to provide a practitioner's view of how we can think about this data and move research into practice.

Reflections for Those Trying to Establish Academic Community Partnerships in the Post-Atlanta Era

The brutal killing of six working-class women of Asian descent on March 16, 2021 in Atlanta, Georgia brought a national spotlight to the kind of racism that Asian Americans have experienced their whole lives. From the beginning of Asian American history, which began with Chinese railroad workers in the mid-1800s, Asian Americans have had to swallow their experiences of racism for mere survival. The complicated history of the Asian American experience, the differences in migration patterns, and the unacknowledged history of imperialism and colonialism in Asia that spurred much of Asian migration, has finally begun to surface in the mainstream American consciousness, challenging America to broaden its understanding of what it means to be a "racial minority" in this country and what it means to be resilient despite the trauma of migration and displacement from one's home country.

Within this reinvigorated and renewed fight for justice that has become a national movement for Asian Americans, research and data have a role. We argue that there is even more urgency for research and data to be community-driven and prioritized. People on the ground, doing the work, see the emerging issues. New problems require new ways of thinking. This is a moment to encourage and challenge researchers to devise creative ways of using research to address community-identified issues and for traditional funding mechanisms to adapt to these changing needs if they, too, want to be responsive.

As a funding agency, we ask the NIH to re-think what it considers "expertise" in community-engaged research and accountability measures. First, we have seen examples of experienced researchers with strong NIH biosketches who have poor community engagement skills. Their approach to community engagement risks damaging the relationship between academia and the community and producing poorer quality data. If these researchers are not able to engage the community properly, they may produce data, but it is unlikely that it will be actionable data for communities. Second, we have seen examples of researchers who say they are doing "community engaged research" but, in actuality, they are using communities for their individual research agenda without investing in a real give-back and mutual benefit for the community. Merely asking a community partner to translate a survey is not community engaged research.

ADAPT community partners are extremely research savvy. Because of their experiences, they are better able to recognize researchers who truly understand the mutual benefits of community engaged research. Their experience in ADAPT has also built their capacity to know how to use research and data strategically to support community needs. Some of the organizations in ADAPT are using this moment to challenge traditional models and measures used in research, such as health behavior research, which many community practitioners say are built and normed on Western models of thinking about wellness and resilience.

Community-based agencies have always been at the forefront of fighting for a most equitable, just, and humane system that serves its constituents, and for ADAPT partners, in particular, much of that fight is for culturally and linguistically appropriate services that are community-based and community-led. They want actionable data. Actionable data is data that communities can use to support their work, that they can present to government and philanthropic funds, and they want written reports that are not just privy to the peer-review world. If they are co-creators of the knowledge, they want to co-create publicly accessible reports, written in lay language that they can put on their websites and social media. Academic researchers and community partners are learning to set up databases that are jointly owned by the researcher and the community so that communities can access the data.

In this new era, we want to challenge academics to re-think their roles in society if they want to continue to be relevant. Should research continue its old narrative that its sole purpose is for generalizable knowledge? Is there a role for research in advocacy and activism in ways that bring actionable data to communities and still preserve the rigor of research? Without accountability measures for academics to deliver actionable data for communities, do communities run the risk of communities being used by academics? If data is not actionable, academics on the other hand can still benefit. They can get papers published, build their CV, and work towards promotion. For academic researchers to stay relevant in this changing political environment, it requires courage.

While this is a difficult and painful moment, it is not without hope. If the academic community can learn how to listen, respect, and honor the lived experience and community partners as equal experts in their own right, then the outlook is bright. If, however, academics continue to cling to old ways of thinking, doing, and knowing, the research enterprise is at risk of becoming irrelevant. We need to find ways to use research and data that can meaningfully and authentically represent the diversity of lived experiences, without just reducing a person's experience to a number Reducing people's experiences to a number, inhibits re-building responsive, humane, and caring systems that are flexible and adaptable to local communities.

Finally, those who have been involved in anti-racist, racial justice, racial liberatory work for decades and those who are new to this work have a responsibility to lean into their growing edge. For ADAPT, our growing edge is to reach outside of Chinatown, which we have already done with other Asian communities, and to reach out to Black communities, where there has been historical tension. For ADAPT to do this work, we have begun to collaborate with Integrating

Underrepresented Populations in Research, a component of Tufts CTSI. This will create opportunities for co-learning, new forms of collaboration, and ultimately, racial healing and reconciliation.

References

1. Rubin CL, Allukian N, Wang X, Ghosh S, Huang CC, Wang J, Brugge D, Wong JB, Mark S, Dong S, Koch-Weser S, Parsons SK, Leslie LK, Freund KM (2014) "We make the path by walking it": building an academic community partnership with Boston Chinatown. Prog Community Health Partnersh 8(3):353–363. https://doi.org/10.1353/cpr.2014.0046
2. Liu M (2020) Forever struggle: activism, identity, & survival in Boston's Chinatown, 1880–2018. Activism, identity, and survival in Boston's Chinatown, 1880–2018. University of Massachusetts Press, Amherst
3. Burns R, Espinola R, Yu L (2018) The Chinese exclusion act. PBS. https://www.pbs.org/wgbh/americanexperience/films/chinese-exclusion-act/#film_description
4. Petersen W (1966) Success, Japanese-American style. New York Times
5. Brand D (1987) The new whiz kids: why Asian Americans are doing so well, and what it costs them. Time 130(9)
6. Metropolitan Area Planning Council (2020) Chinatown master plan 2020. https://www.mapc.org/resource-library/chinatown-master-plan-2020/

Chapter 21
Stakeholder Engagement in Predictive Model Development for Clinical Decision Support

Denise H. Daudelin

Abstract This chapter describes a study to develop a practical tool to help patients and their clinicians choose which type of knee osteoarthritis treatment would be best for the patient. This tool, which is based on highly technical predictive models, would identify the most appropriate treatment option for a specific patient by taking into account a patient's characteristics, clinical condition, and other variables that patients, their families, and their clinicians consider when making such choices. It was important to ensure that both patients and clinicians had confidence in the tool's utility and feasibility. We describe the ways in which patients and clinicians were involved in the study and some of the challenges we encountered to ensure these groups gained the information they needed to participate and trust in the value of their contributions.

Keywords Stakeholder engagement in methods research · Treatment decision making · Predictive model development · Decision support tool

Stakeholder engagement is becoming a more common component of comparative effectiveness research, but it is less common in research that involves evidence synthesis, integration, dissemination, and application. The literature pertaining to stakeholder engagement in methods research is relatively sparse [1]. We conducted a methodological study to develop a decision-making tool for patients and clinicians that would help guide decisions about the available treatment options for knee osteoarthritis. This tool depends on predictive models. While predictive models are highly technical, we were interested in populating a model that incorporated scientific information as well as the perspectives and preferences of patients, their family members, and clinicians. To achieve this objective, we included stakeholder participation in study design, development of predictive models, and use of the models in

D. H. Daudelin (✉)
Tufts Clinical and Translational Science Institute; Institute for Clinical Research and Health Policy Studies, Tufts Medical Center, Boston, MA, USA
e-mail: ddaudelin@tuftsmedicalcenter.org

© The Author(s), under exclusive license to Springer Nature Switzerland AG 2022
D. Lerner et al. (eds.), *Broadly Engaged Team Science in Clinical and Translational Research*, https://doi.org/10.1007/978-3-030-83028-1_21

creating a decision support tool. Involvement of stakeholders in this methodological study presented some challenges but resulted in a decision support tool which reflected the clinical outcomes most important to patients and clinicians.

When incorporated into shared patient-clinician decision making, decision support tools or decision aids have been found to improve patient knowledge and to help patients clarify their personal values and make value-congruent decisions with their clinicians [2, 3]. In severe osteoarthritis, shared patient-clinician decision making is central to choosing between non-surgical treatments and surgical total knee replacement (TKR) as a preference-sensitive care choice. Although quantification of the harms and benefits of the options in decision support tools is typically based on aggregate data, in this project we set out to develop a decision support tool that would be targeted to individual-specific characteristics by using predictive models. To make those models relevant to patients with knee osteoarthritis and their clinicians, and to maximize the usefulness and uptake of the tool, we involved patients, family members, patient advocates, specialists, generalists, allied health clinicians, and researchers as stakeholders in model development.

For this project, we developed the Knee Osteoarthritis Mathematical Equipoise Tool (KOMET) to provide patient-specific decision support for shared decision making when choosing between non-surgical treatments and surgical TKR. We engaged stakeholders in an iterative process to seek their knowledge, experience, and values regarding treatment decision making and incorporated their perspectives to ensure that the predictive models were relevant to patient-clinician decision-making [4]. This chapter summarizes key methods, considerations, and lessons learned through engaging stakeholders in the process of developing the predictive models. Stakeholder involvement in study design and development and testing of the decision support tool are reported elsewhere [5, 6].

Methods

Developing predictive models involves first identifying the health outcome of interest and the question to be answered. Next, a database of patient related data variables, including the outcomes of treatments, is created. Stakeholders determine which among the many variables may be important and useful in predicting the outcome of interest. Those variables are used to develop predictive mathematical models and their performance in predicting the outcome is tested. The model is then refined to reach a final version with good predictive performance that is meaningful to clinicians and patients for decision-making and uses data that is feasible to collect. Finally, as in this study, the model is embedded in a computer software application which uses patient information to display patient-specific outcome predictions.

To develop KOMET's predictive models for clinical outcomes of TKR and of non-surgical treatments, we created a consolidated database with treatment outcomes of severe knee osteoarthritis from a variety of clinical study and registry data. Model variables were selected based on conversations with patients and clinicians and on an analysis of variables' contributions to our? models' predictive performance. These variables? were then incorporated into decision support software prototypes that were pilot tested with stakeholders, clinicians, and patients [5, 6]. The project was conducted between January 2014 and December 2017.

Stakeholder Outreach

Stakeholders were selected to represent the range of individuals or groups responsible for, or affected by, health- and health care-related decisions about knee osteoarthritis treatments [7]. Two stakeholder panels, one composed of patients, families, and patient advocates and another of clinicians and researchers, were created to structure and facilitate engagement. Both panels met in person quarterly between January 2014 and February 2017 and equal compensation was provided for patients, families, and clinicians.

The patient stakeholder panel included individuals who were: (1) at risk for knee osteoarthritis due to osteoarthritis in other joints, (2) actively considering treatment options for their knee osteoarthritis, and (3) previously treated with TKR for severe knee osteoarthritis. The seven patient stakeholder panel members were identified through clinicians, knee osteoarthritis researchers, and the Arthritis Foundation referrals. We sought viewpoints from patients actively considering their treatment options as well as from those who recently received TKR. We selected patient advocates with a broad perspective on the needs of people with arthritis and patients' family members with insight into the impact of the family environment on decision making. Some of the patients had participated in knee osteoarthritis research previously and had experience providing the type of patient reported outcomes data we planned to use in model development.

The seven clinician and researcher panel stakeholders were recruited among local primary care, orthopedic, and rheumatology clinicians and researchers. The clinician panel included two rheumatologists, two primary care physicians, two orthopedic surgeons, and one physical therapist. Both of the rheumatologists and one of the orthopedic surgeons were also researchers themselves and were able to represent the researcher perspective. Each type of physician was selected based on experience either treating patients within a particular setting and stage of the disease or conducting related research studies.

Building Capacity for Full Stakeholder Participation

Research team members participated in quarterly in-person panel meetings by facilitating discussions and providing education on study methods. They introduced patient stakeholders to decision support model development to ensure that stakeholders had sufficient knowledge about the modeling process, confidence in their ability to contribute to the activity, and were comfortable providing their perspective. Stakeholders received materials to review in advance of panel meetings and had the opportunity to ask questions about knee osteoarthritis treatment and outcomes in order to feel better prepared for their role in the project.

During training, patient stakeholders were led through an exercise on developing a straightforward model predicting height and weight to illustrate the steps in model development and help them understand the value of contributing their perspective to the model development process (Fig. 21.1). Clinician training included a discussion of decision support research and decision support examples such as using statin medications for preventing cardiovascular events. Patient and clinician panel meetings were conducted separately so that the content and terminology addressed the interests and learning needs of the members. The study team provided a bridge between the groups sharing perspectives and concerns. We facilitated discussions about what mattered most to patients and clinicians involved in the shared decision-making process and how it should shape the design of the decision support tool. The intent was to share with stakeholders the successes and challenges of the project and to learn from stakeholders if the project's direction and resulting decision support tool were addressing stakeholder needs.

Stakeholder engagement around the goals of the study began with one-on-one conversations during the planning of the research project and continued once the study was underway with moderated panel discussions. Specifically, we asked stakeholders to consider the question, *"If an adult with knee osteoarthritis is presented with medical and surgical treatment options, what decision support could be*

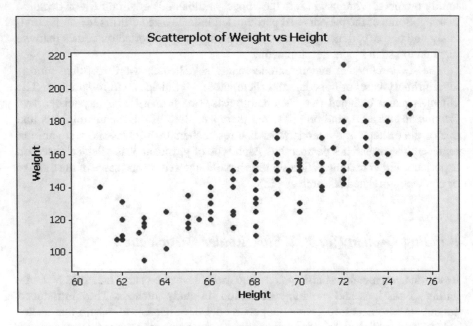

Fig. 21.1 Example of model development used in patient stakeholder training selection of study questions and outcomes

provided at the point of care that the clinician and patient can use to understand the patient-specific predicted outcomes of importance to the patient?" During these discussions, stakeholders described the importance of knee osteoarthritis treatments that alleviate pain and return people to their desired level of physical functioning. This confirmed and clarified the selection of knee pain and overall functional health status as outcomes of interest for the development of predictive models and decision support. In addition, stakeholders discussed their experiences in making knee osteo-arthritis treatment decisions and pain and function related factors that influenced these preference-sensitive decisions. These discussions also included other treat-ment considerations such as risk factors, family support, rehabilitation, employment and retirement, and socioeconomic issues. Patient and clinician panels also were asked how factors such as the joint replacement lifespan and the impact of multiple comorbidities affected considerations about the timing and desirability of knee replacement. The responses to these questions informed study outcome selection, the creation of the study database, and the development of the predictive models.

Predictive Model Development

The database created for development of the predictive models for two key out-comes of knee replacement surgery, pain and function, combined four data sets, as well as stakeholder input about which of the many potential variables should be retained for further analysis. To rank the variables, stakeholders rated each vari-able's importance in determining pain and functional outcomes (ranging from not at all important to very important) and perceived feasibility of collecting the necessary data (ranging from very easy to very hard). This process helped to prioritize which variables to include or exclude in the models.

Additionally, because the knee pain and overall function predictive models would be based on patient-reported pain and function survey instrument data, we sought patient and clinician feedback on the meaningfulness of the various assess-ment questions and omissions of important aspects of pain and function. We asked what future period they would want to consider as they made a treatment decision. Would they want to consider their pain and function in 3 months, 6 months, 1 year, or 2 years? We also sought input on topics not addressed by these tools such as the rehabilitation period after total knee replacement.

Throughout the project, we asked stakeholders how frequently, at what point in the disease progression, and in which settings (home, clinician office) they might expect to use the predicted outcomes in decision-making. We also asked patient and clinician stakeholders about the feasibility of using an electronic versus paper-based decision support tool and the usefulness of tracking predictions over time as the patient's health status changed. These questions recognize the potential influence of the social context and illness trajectory on decision-making.

Results

Stakeholder Engagement

Seventy-one percent (5/7) of the patient stakeholders and all of the clinician and researcher stakeholders remained engaged throughout the project. Two patient stakeholders discontinued their participation for undetermined reasons in the last year of the study after the models were developed.

Selection of Study Questions and Outcomes

Stakeholders strongly supported using both the knee pain and functional outcomes in patients' decision-making processes about TKR or non-surgical treatment. Our choice of outcomes, improvement in physical function and pain relief, reflects these as the two primary concerns of the patients and clinicians. Stakeholders and clinicians described the importance of pain relief in order to improve physical and emotional functioning. While discussions with stakeholders revealed that considerations of treatment outcomes were nuanced and that pain and function were deeply interconnected, separate models for pain and physical function were developed to allow patients to consider each dimension separately.

Stakeholders also discussed a range of other outcomes and considerations that they believed should be included in a decision support tool. These included cost, rehabilitation considerations, lost time at work, future quality of life, and risks. Though, due to project scope limitations, we were unable to incorporate these additional considerations, these attributes could be considered for future model revisions.

Predictive Model Development

Stakeholder engagement influenced the development of the modeling database and the predictive model. Stakeholders contributed insights into the meaningfulness and interpretation of pain and function survey questions, the importance of postoperative factors in decision-making, and the ease of collection of variables. Clinician and patient stakeholders provided input on the model's variables, the clinical significance and feasibility of collecting the variables, and the results of the predictive models. Candidate primary and interaction variables included in the selection process were those considered important, plausible, and easily and reliably provided by stakeholders. Once the model was developed and the computer software was being designed, the research team and stakeholders decided that many of the variables under consideration were burdensome to collect or difficult to capture in a consistent manner. We were able to respond by removing these variables without diminishing the performance characteristics of the model. Once the models were developed, stakeholders contributed extensively to the design of the decision support application's user interface and features [6].

Expanding Stakeholder Engagement in Methodological Research

Patient, clinician, and researcher stakeholders played an integral part in this methodological project to develop mathematical models that predict patient-specific outcomes of treatment options for knee osteoarthritis and a decision-support program. While stakeholders are increasingly involved in Comparative Effectiveness Research, the role of stakeholders in studies that involve using expert knowledge to develop innovative research *methods*, such as this study, is less common. We addressed the fundamental considerations given stakeholder engagement in other types of research with an emphasis on educating stakeholders on the project methods and promoting stakeholder beliefs about the importance, value, and impact of their involvement [8]. Insights learned from stakeholder participation shaped the development of the predictive models.

A challenge involved in engaging stakeholders in methodological research is to ensure they have sufficient research training and feel prepared to contribute their perspectives when decisions regarding the methodology are being made [9]. To accomplish this, we provided patient and non-researcher clinician stakeholders with an overview of the predictive modeling process using straightforward examples and sought their input on specific questions about the selection of the outcomes and model variables, and the usefulness of model output. We also structured panel meetings to address topics in which stakeholders believed they needed additional information. For patients this included providing information about current advances in knee osteoarthritis treatment, rehabilitation, and research. For clinicians, we facilitated conversations with peers on pain management and other osteoarthritis therapies.

Maintaining engagement of all clinician and most patient stakeholders throughout the project required flexibility in planning study activities. Patient stakeholders often needed to join meetings by phone or provide their views outside of the panel meeting time when their health or family commitments prevented travel. While two patient stakeholders did not continue in the final year of the project, all stakeholders actively contributed to model development. Clinician and researcher stakeholders often had difficulty attending meetings due to clinical commitments requiring briefer lunchtime sessions or individual conversations with the study team.

Our experience engaging stakeholders in developing the predictive models illustrate both benefits and challenges of stakeholder engagement in methodological research. Stakeholders provided insight into the selection of outcomes and model variables thereby ensuring that the study team was including those outcomes most important to patients with severe knee osteoarthritis and not requiring a burdensome level of data collection. While we focused on those outcomes of importance to stakeholders, the selection of outcomes was limited by the availability of data for model development and the study timeframe. Patient stakeholders were interested in outcomes not represented in our modeling dataset and suggested that the predicted pain and function numerical scale composite outcomes available in the dataset be translated to important functional activities such as gardening or climbing stairs. This raises the issue of incorporating meaningful patient-centered outcomes into study design. More in-depth engagement of stakeholders when selecting databases on which to base the models could have revealed that additional data sources were needed. This also illustrates the importance of reconsidering whether numerical outputs should be the only method for the decision support or if there are other options to better address patients for whom the numerical outputs are not as meaningful.

In addition to the limitation above, our project focus included only the benefits of each treatment decision despite the importance of considering both benefit and harm [10]. More thorough stakeholder engagement initially would have allowed us to address both the need for meaningful functional descriptions of outcomes and potential harms in the design of the decision support.

Methodological research like this has the opportunity to benefit from stakeholder engagement by ensuring that the perspectives of those most impacted by the results are involved in study design, execution, and dissemination. While additional planning and investments in maintaining stakeholder knowledge and trust may be needed, they are offset by the valuable insights gained. Although there is a tradition of stakeholder engagement in clinical and community research, it has been less common in methodological research. We think such input greatly benefited our project and we hope our experience informs other researchers on the role of stakeholders in methodological studies.

Acknowledgements The authors wish to thank our patient and clinician stakeholders for their valuable contributions and guidance: Debra Band-Entrup, Kathie Bernstein, Melvin Bernstein, Jaclyn Chu, Deane Felter, William Harvey, Helen Herzer, Cristina MacDonald, Vincent MacDonald, Susan Nesci, John Richmond, Kimberly Schelling, Eric Smith, and Steven Vlad.

Research reported in this chapter was funded through a Patient-Centered Outcomes Research Institute (PCORI) Award (ME-1306-02327). The views, statements, and opinions presented in this report are solely the responsibility of the author(s) and do not necessarily represent the views of the Patient-Centered Outcomes Research Institute (PCORI), its Board of Governors or Methodology Committee.

References

1. Concannon TW, Fuster M, Saunders T, Patel K, Wong JB, Leslie LK, Lau J (2014) A systematic review of stakeholder engagement in comparative effectiveness and patient-centered outcomes research. J Gen Intern Med 29(12):1692–1701. https://doi.org/10.1007/s11606-014-2878-x
2. Bozic KJ, Belkora J, Chan V, Youm J, Zhou T, Dupaix J, Bye AN, Braddock CH 3rd, Chenok KE, Huddleston JI 3rd (2013) Shared decision making in patients with osteoarthritis of the hip

and knee: results of a randomized controlled trial. J Bone Joint Surg Am 95(18):1633–1639. https://doi.org/10.2106/JBJS.M.00004

3. Stacey D, Legare F, Lewis K, Barry MJ, Bennett CL, Eden KB, Holmes-Rovner M, Llewellyn-Thomas H, Lyddiatt A, Thomson R, Trevena L (2017) Decision aids for people facing health treatment or screening decisions. Cochrane Database Syst Rev 4:CD001431. https://doi.org/10.1002/14651858.CD001431.pub5

4. Deverka PA, Lavallee DC, Desai PJ, Esmail LC, Ramsey SD, Veenstra DL, Tunis SR (2012) Stakeholder participation in comparative effectiveness research: defining a framework for effective engagement. J Comp Eff Res 1(2):181–194. https://doi.org/10.2217/cer.12.7

5. Selker HP, Daudelin DH, Ruthazer R, Kwong M, Lorenzana RC, Hannon DJ, Wong JB, Kent DM, Terrin N, Moreno-Koehler AD, McAlindon TE (2019) The use of patient-specific equipoise to support shared decision-making for clinical care and enrollment into clinical trials. J Clin Transl Sci 3(1):27–36. https://doi.org/10.1017/cts.2019.380

6. Daudelin DH, Ruthazer R, Kwong M, Lorenzana RC, Hannon DJ, Kent DM, McAlindon TE, Terrin N, Wong JB, Selker HP (2020) Stakeholder engagement in methodological research: development of a clinical decision support tool. J Clin Transl Sci 4(2):133–140. https://doi.org/10.1017/cts.2019.443

7. Concannon TW, Meissner P, Grunbaum JA, McElwee N, Guise J-M, Santa J, Conway PH, Daudelin D, Morrato EH, Leslie LK (2012) A new taxonomy for stakeholder engagement in patient-centered outcomes research. J Gen Intern Med 27(8):985–991. https://doi.org/10.1007/s11606-012-2037-1

8. Cukor D, Cohen LM, Cope EL, Ghahramani N, Hedayati SS, Hynes DM, Shah VO, Tentori F, Unruh M, Bobelu J, Cohen S, Dember LM, Faber T, Fischer MJ, Gallardo R, Germain MJ, Ghahate D, Grote N, Hartwell L, Heagerty P, Kimmel PL, Kutner N, Lawson S, Marr L, Nelson RG, Porter AC, Sandy P, Struminger BB, Subramanian L, Weisbord S, Young B, Mehrotra R (2016) Patient and other stakeholder engagement in patient-centered outcomes research institute funded studies of patients with kidney diseases. Clin J Am Soc Nephrol 11(9):1703–1712. https://doi.org/10.2215/CJN.09780915

9. Forsythe LP, Frank L, Walker KO, Anise A, Wegener N, Weisman H, Hunt G, Beal A (2015) Patient and clinician views on comparative effectiveness research and engagement in research. J Comp Eff Res 4(1):11–25. https://doi.org/10.2217/cer.14.52

10. Katz JN (2015) Parachutes and preferences--a trial of knee replacement. N Engl J Med 373(17):1668–1669. https://doi.org/10.1056/NEJMe1510312

Part IV
Creating an Institutional Environment of Support for Broadly Engaged Team Science

Chapter 22
Research Administration Practices for Proposal Development and Post-Award Management of Stakeholders and Community Participants

Carol Seidel

Abstract Using non-academic or non-scientific stakeholder partners in research studies requires coordination with research administration to ensure proposal and post-award funding requirements are met and managed in a way that is compliant with funder and institutional policies. Stakeholders may be patients, caregivers, clinicians, researchers, advocacy groups, professional societies, business, or policy makers. Grant funding agencies have developed proposal guidelines and policies that are often academic-centric and not easily applicable to the stakeholder role, although some are beginning to recognize the need for specific processes and modify the guidance for managing these important collaborations. In this chapter, we will review key areas where clarity is often needed for research administrators and the Principal Investigators (PI) when developing research funding proposals and planning for post-award start-up of projects that include stakeholder engagement. Each academic institution has different processes and policies, and each funding agency and specific programs within may have different requirements. These are often updated and should be reviewed carefully at the time of proposal and award to have the best information possible for successful funding and administrative compliance.

Keywords Non-scientific stakeholder · Community stakeholders · Stakeholder involvement · Stakeholder biosketch · Engaging stakeholders

Involving stakeholders in research projects is an important step in broadly engaged team science to help with priority setting and ensure the research is aligned with the needs of those most impacted. Using non-academic or non-scientific community

C. Seidel (✉)
Institute for Clinical Research and Health Policy Studies, Tufts Medical Center,
Boston, MA, USA
e-mail: cseidel@tuftsmedicalcenter.org

© The Author(s), under exclusive license to Springer Nature
Switzerland AG 2022
D. Lerner et al. (eds.), *Broadly Engaged Team Science in Clinical and Translational Research*, https://doi.org/10.1007/978-3-030-83028-1_22

stakeholders in research studies requires coordination with research administration to ensure proposal and post-award funding requirements are met and managed in a way that is compliant with funder and institutional policies. Stakeholders may be patients, caregivers, clinicians, researchers, advocacy groups, professional societies, business, or policy makers. If they do not typically work on research projects, stakeholders may not have in place the necessary certifications, descriptions, or organizational policies [1]. Grant funding agencies have developed proposal guidelines and policies that are often academic-centric and not easily applicable to certain stakeholder roles, although some are beginning to recognize the need for specific processes and guidance for managing all of these important collaborations. The Patient-Centered Outcomes Research Institute (PCORI) has been a leader in making stakeholder engagement a requirement and in the development and dissemination of proposal guidelines and best practices that respond to the variation in experiences. The Agency for Healthcare Research and Quality (AHRQ) and National Institutes of Health (NIH) are also recognizing the importance of engaging stakeholders in the research process, but they have few specific processes for managing these varied roles, and research administrators at the institutional level need to work closely with these partners to ensure federal funding requirements are being met.

In this chapter, I review key areas where clarity is often needed for research administrators and the Principal Investigators (PI) when developing research funding proposals and planning for post-award start-up of projects that include broad stakeholder engagement. Each academic institution has different processes and policies, and each funding agency and specific programs may have different requirements. These are often updated and should be reviewed carefully at the time of proposal and award to have the best information possible for successful funding and administrative compliance.

Determining Research Roles and Requirements for Budget Development

The PI and research team first must determine the need for stakeholders during development of the research proposal and execution of a funded study. Stakeholders may engage with researchers at several different levels of involvement. Understanding the activity level and sharing this information with the research administrator will help inform how to plan for compensation and execute formal agreements for engagement. Table 22.1, adapted from the PCORI framework, provides some examples of the spectrum of increasing levels of engagement in research [2].

After considering the level of activity required, the next decision point in stakeholder-engaged research is identifying the actual role the stakeholder will have on the research project. Stakeholder involvement can range from shared project leadership to general project support. Each level of stakeholder involvement has specific proposal and budget requirements when applying to agencies such as PCORI or the NIH. Additionally, these roles and responsibilities provide a basis for developing a work plan, project timetable, and other important grant proposal elements.

Table 22.2 outlines five typical levels of stakeholder involvement, from the research administration perspective, associated roles and responsibilities to the project, along with specific examples of proposal and budgetary requirements [3, 4]. These requirements may change and should be reviewed with the funding announcement and funding agency policies currently in place.

Table 22.1 Examples of engagement in research

Engagement activity	Role	Example
Inform	Informing	Communicating plans to patient community
Consult	Consulting on decisions	Offering advice, opinions, feedback
Collaborate	Deciding or acting together	Joint decisions solicited and taking actions jointly
Stakeholder directed	Encouraging independent initiatives	Leading patient/caregiver/organization research

Table 22.2 Proposal development by stakeholder role

Stakeholder role	Responsibility	Proposal requirements	Budget structure

Shared PI or investigator	Works with the PI as key personnel in the scientific development or execution of a project for a specific percentage of time. Maybe employed or affiliated with the applicant/grantee organization or another organization	Biosketch for key personnel
		  NIH eRA commons ID (for AHRQ or NIH funding)
		  Personal statement reflecting leadership role in project.
		If a subaward/consortium:
		  Statement of intent with scope of work, assurances and certifications signed by organization*
		  Federal Wide Assurance (FWA) for human subjects research, DUNS number, and EIN number*
		  Budget and budget justification
		  Letter of support to PI
		  Information on facilities and resources
		  Indirect cost (F&A) rate agreement or basis for rate.
		  Human subjects research training if applicable
			*Subcontract budget with specific budget line items for salary, fringe, travel costs, other expenses, F&A
			Budget justification

(continued)

Table 22.2 (continued)

Stakeholder role	Responsibility	Proposal requirements	Budget structure
Individual consultant	Provides professional advice or services for a fee, but typically not as an employee of the engaging party. May be key personnel engaging in research questions or in core portions of the research study	Biosketch if key personnel with personal statement reflecting consulting role and relevant experience Letter of support from consultant to PI Human subjects research training completed if applicable If individual is working on behalf of a community agency justification should include intention to obtain a FWA*	Specific budget line item included under consultants. Budget justification should include clear statement about what the consultant will be doing, how often and for how much.
Individual advisor or member of advisory board	Provides consultative and expert advice to PIs, but is typically not considered key personnel May include assistance or feedback in following examples: Development of surveys and other data collection activities Suggestions regarding recruitment Interpretation of findings Dissemination activities Support the project work May help with recruitment.	Letter of support indicating purpose of the advisory role or board membership, how often they will be engaged, what kind of input they will provide, and specific expertise that they bring to the project.	Budget justification should include payment to advisor as a specific research expense. In some instances, PIs may wish to include costs incurred by the advisor in the budget as a specific research expense. (e.g., honoraria, travel expenses, childcare coverage, meeting expenses, etc.)

(continued)

Table 22.2   (continued)

Stakeholder role	Responsibility	Proposal requirements	Budget structure
Non-profit/ community organization support or advisors	Development of surveys Suggestions regarding recruitment Interpretation of findings Dissemination activities Support the project work May help with recruitment Focus groups with community members Open community forum to discuss project	Letter of support describing the community organization and its role in the project. Subaward/consortium agreement is not needed if the organization is not engaging in research, but providing a service	In some instances, PIs may wish to include costs incurred by the community organization in the budget as a specific research expense. (e.g., honoraria, travel expenses, childcare coverage, meeting expenses, etc.)

*Assurances and Identifiers Definitions and Links:
- **Statement of Intent with Assurances and Certifications**: The prime grant recipient is responsible for ensuring all required terms and conditions flow down to a subrecipient, and these terms are included in the subaward agreement. The Federal Demonstration Project (www.thefdp.org) is an association of federal agencies, academic research institutions with administrative, faculty and technical representation, and research policy organizations that work to streamline the administration of federally sponsored research. The FDP has developed standardized forms and templates to use between FDP member institutions as well as non-FDP organizations. These templates are updated as needed to include federal requirements.
- **Federalwide Assurance (FWA)**: If the researcher/consultant is working on behalf of a community agency or organization and the federally funded project involves human subjects, the budget justification should include an intention to obtain a Federal-wide Assurance (FWA) as part of the subcontract. The FWA is a way for an institution, such as a community center, to say they agree to follow governmental research rules. An FWA ensures research participant safety and confidentiality.https://www.hhs.gov/ohrp/register-irbs-and-obtain-fwas/fwas/fwa-protection-of-human-subjecct/index.html
- **DUNS number**: A **DUNS number** is a unique nine-character number used to identify your organization. The federal government uses the DUNS number to track how federal money is allocated.https://www.test.grants.gov/applicants/organization-registration/step-1-obtain-duns-number.html
- **EIN number:** An Employer Identification Number (EIN) is also known as a Federal Tax Identification Number and is used to identify a business entity.https://www.irs.gov/businesses/small-businesses-self-employed/apply-for-an-employer-identification-number-ein-online

Planning for Compensation

PCORI published a guide, *Compensation Framework for Engaged Research Partners,* which provides guidelines for compensating stakeholders for their roles on sponsored research projects [2]. Research partners may be individuals or organizations. While the PCORI document provides specifics for its program applicants, there are certain compensation guidelines we tend to follow within our institution.

Generally, compensation of stakeholders should reflect the level of expertise, commitment, responsibility, the type of work involved, and the degree of participation expected, in line with other members of the research team. Within research teams, pay scales may vary widely among professionals based on local market trends for specific roles, education levels, and years of experience. At the highest level, stakeholders who are acting as engaged research partners and who share in making decisions relating to the research should be compensated consistent with other professionals on the team. At the less active end of the continuum may be patients acting as engaged research partners who inform others, and in these cases, honoraria or in-kind vouchers may be more reflective of the value made to the research endeavor. There is no set guideline on appropriate rates to use per activity. The PI, in discussion with the research administrator, can use base compensation levels of individuals, funding announcement guidelines and budget restrictions, and local or institutional usual rates to determine what is appropriate for the project and the individual.

Compensation models should allow for some flexibility, such as allowing engaged stakeholders to choose to decline compensation given restrictions that may apply to them (e.g., restrictions of their employers or affiliated organizations). Please note that stakeholders should be notified that all income, regardless of amount, is subject to relevant tax laws and regulations. Current information can be found at www.irs.gov

Planning a Proposal Budget that Includes Stakeholders

The optimal budget amount and tools needed are dependent on whether the work will be done by an individual or through an organization. Using the decisions made for the engagement activity, stakeholder role, and compensation plans, the PI, in discussion with the research administrator, should follow the format of the funding agency guidance to build the budget and required supporting materials for a proposal. Requirements can change cycle to cycle for funding opportunities, so it is important to review current guidance for stakeholder engagement, budget rules or restrictions, and documentation.

Stakeholders may have different budgetary needs than the research team. For instance, to allow full engagement in the project, they may need help paying for transportation, technology assistance, caregiver assistance, and the like. Where allowed by the funding agency, costs like these should be considered for inclusion. When the project is funded, the research administrator and PI should work through the institutional processes to put in place a subaward or subcontract, consulting agreement, or billing agreement with the stakeholder organization or individual at time of award or engagement. Each instrument has different requirements for planning the budget.

1. If *working with an organization as part of the research team*, a subaward including a detailed budget and required contract materials will be needed. The budget should include all personnel costs (including salary and fringe benefits), other expenses and Facilities and Administrative Costs (F&A), following the policies of the institution and funding agency. Effort of key personnel and other staff should reflect the estimated time and expertise required to do the work. Develop a budget justification and a scope of work that describes in detail the work of the contracting organization or individual. If the institution does not have a federally negotiated rate for fringe benefits or F&A, NIH will allow 10% based on modified total direct costs. PCORI allows up to 40% indirect costs but requires documentation for the basis of the rate requested. A signed statement of intent with organizational address and identifiers, budget information, and scope of work that mirror the project budget and justification will be needed. It is helpful to have an administrative contact to work with at the contracting organization, in addition to the collaborator. This helps to identify early issues regarding compliance or special organizational requirements impacting the project and avoid delays in agreements and the sign-off on a statement of intent.

2. If working with *an individual consultant*, compensation should be planned for the level of work and expertise of the consultant and the time commitment expected. This can be based on an hourly rate, daily rate, or flat rate agreed upon for the effort and/or deliverable work product. How to determine appropriate consulting rates is deliberately vague and "reasonable rates" are defined as what a prudent person would pay in the conduct of a competitive business. It may help to reach out to the Bureau of Labor Statistics, professional or trade associations, or search online for compensation surveys for particular expertise [5]. A detailed scope of work including projected period of performance and amount of time required will be needed for the budget justification and establishing an agreement post-award.

3. If working with an *advisory board member or a community organization*, include these costs under "other expense" for honoraria (or in-kind payments in lieu of compensation), and other expenses related to participation in the project, including travel expenses, materials, meeting expenses and the like. The justification should include detailed information about the role and the basis for cost.

Preparing Biosketches for Key Personnel

Biosketches *are* used to highlight each individual's qualifications for a specific role in a proposed project and are required for key personnel roles. The form template, particularly through NIH, may present challenges to certain stakeholders as typically they are geared to scientific accomplishments and publications. It may be unclear for community stakeholders how best to complete this form and they may be concerned about how reviewers will receive their answers in sections related to education, positions held, contribution to science, and publications. To ease these concerns, PCORI has developed a separate stakeholder biosketch template geared to non-scientist stakeholders. In both NIH and PCORI biosketch formats, there is a section for a personal statement, where the stakeholder should highlight their relevant background to the project and the role, describing previous advocacy, advisory, or stakeholder roles, experience with the condition being studied, or employment or education that prepared them for collaboration. Frequently, the stakeholder has no peer-reviewed scientific publications, and in that case, it is acceptable to indicate "none." They may note non peer-reviewed published materials such as educational materials, patient engagement materials, or other experience such as videos, blogs, etc. For the contribution to science section, the stakeholder may highlight other research projects or subject matter advocacy they have been involved in that contributed to scientific understanding of a problem. This may also be left blank. Reviewers understand that stakeholders hold a different type of experience and expertise than researchers and do not expect the biosketches to be similar.

Letter of Support

It is often required or recommended that stakeholders include a letter of support for the proposal describing their enthusiasm for participation, their role and that of their organization, and the terms of their involvement, including proposed dates and compensation as discussed. This letter should be addressed to the PI or team and written on organization letterhead, if available. It may help for consistency and clarity for the PI or research team member to draft a template of this letter for community stakeholders to personalize.

Human Subjects Concerns

Investigators and all key personnel who will be involved in the design or conduct of NIH-funded human subjects research must fulfill the Protection of Human Subjects education requirement. Training modules are typically available through the prime academic institution's Institutional Review Board (IRB). Often these training modules are geared only toward those with research experience, although options are being developed for community stakeholders. For example, the University of Illinois at Chicago's Center for Clinical and Translational Science has developed a program, "CIRTification: Community Involvement in Research Training." CIRTification is designed specifically for community research partners with little or no prior research experience [6].

Practices Continue to Evolve

Practices for grant submissions and funded projects relating to the use of stakeholders in research continues to evolve. It is important for the PI to plan well ahead of the proposal submission to review the guidelines and to begin identifying and incorporating stakeholders in the research. The research administrator or grants specialist at the research institution should be involved early in the process and can assist with understanding agency or organizational requirements, budget and financial management policies, and issues of compliance that need to be vetted in advance of the deadline. A smooth transition from the proposal preparation to activating a funded project can happen with advance planning and attention to the challenges. Involving community stakeholders will ensure that research projects are aligned with the priorities and needs of those most impacted by the research topic. Research Administration departments are learning about this new area at the same time as researchers and it is likely that innovative approaches to engaging stakeholders on research teams will continue to evolve as experience is gained.

References

1. Public policy requirements, objectives and other appropriation mandates (2019). https://grants.nih.gov/grants/policy/nihgps/html5/section_4/4.1_public_policy_requirements_and_objectives.htm
2. Financial compensation of patients, caregivers, and patient/caregiver organizations engaged in PCORI-funded research as engaged research partners (2015). PCORI
3. Burke JG, Jones J, Yonas M, Guizzetti L, Virata MC, Costlow M, Morton SC, Elizabeth M (2013) PCOR, CER, and CBPR: alphabet soup or complementary fields of health research? Clin Transl Sci 6(6):493–496. https://doi.org/10.1111/cts.12064
4. University of Pittsburgh and UPMC Stakeholder Engagement Resource Guide (2015) University of Pittsburgh Comparative Effectiveness Center, Pittsburgh
5. U.S Bureau of Labor Statistics (2019) Overview of BLS wage data by area and occupation. https://www.bls.gov/bls/blswage.htm
6. Using CIRTification. University of Illinois Chicago. https://ccts.uic.edu/tools/cirtification/use/

Chapter 23
Starting Off Right: Supporting Community Involvement in the Evaluation of Research Proposals

Robert Sege and Marguerite Fenwood Hughes

Abstract Tufts Clinical and Translational Science Institute's (CTSI) Stakeholder and Community Engagement (SCE) Program strives to support partnered research that is relevant, understandable, and useful to a variety of stakeholders across the translational spectrum both locally and nationally. This support includes promoting the involvement of stakeholders in all phases of research, beginning with research planning. In this context, every proposal that is submitted to certain Tufts CTSI research grant and graduate training programs must include a stakeholder engagement plan, which is reviewed and rated by a standing committee of our Stakeholder Expert Panel. This chapter describes the infrastructure Tufts CTSI established to perform these critical reviews. We explain the set of proposals that require stakeholder engagement plans, the key elements that must be included in a stakeholder engagement plan, methods for training researchers and reviewers about stakeholder engagement, and finally, the review process itself.

Keywords Tufts CTSI · Stakeholder engagement plan

Tufts Clinical and Translational Science Institute's (CTSI) Stakeholder and Community Engagement (SCE) Program offers services and resources for researchers to meaningfully involve stakeholders and communities in translational research. The objective of the SCE Program is to support partnered research that is relevant, understandable, and useful to a variety of stakeholders across the translational spectrum both locally and nationally. The translational spectrum encompasses five phases of translational research: basic science, pre- clinical research, clinical research, clinical implementation, and public health. Stakeholders of many types can be involved at every translational phase and in all stages of research, beginning with research planning.

R. Sege (✉) · M. F. Hughes
Tufts Clinical and Translational Science Institute, Tufts Medical Center, Boston, MA, USA
e-mail: rsege@tuftsmedicalcenter.org

© The Author(s), under exclusive license to Springer Nature Switzerland AG 2022
D. Lerner et al. (eds.), *Broadly Engaged Team Science in Clinical and Translational Research*, https://doi.org/10.1007/978-3-030-83028-1_23

Tufts CTSI strives for authentic stakeholder-engaged research. Towards that goal, research proposals requesting CTSI funding or graduate student theses submitted in accordance with Tufts CTSI's Program in Clinical and Translational Science graduation requirements, must include a stakeholder engagement plan. These plans are reviewed and scored by a committee of Tufts CTSI Stakeholder Expert Panel. Developing the capacity to include community input into the review and evaluation of CTSI-funded research and training activities required focused attention on the need to develop new capacities among community members, students, and researchers. To develop the needed capacity, a cooperative plan was created by directors from the Tufts CTSI SCE Program, a project manager, community stakeholders, and the Tufts CTSI pilot funding and evaluation teams. This plan now serves as a blueprint for action.

Since its inception, Tufts CTSI has used traditional peer review processes to drive the selection of proposals for competitive funding opportunities. The scientific peer reviewers are primarily responsible for technical reviews that address proposal innovation, importance, and feasibility. However, because peer reviewers may have little background or understanding of stakeholder engagement or may not prioritize the stakeholder engagement plan section in their overall evaluation and scoring of proposals, we developed a specific, parallel procedure for the assessment of the quality of stakeholder engagement plans. First, we assembled a Stakeholder Expert Panel, many of whom have been research participants themselves or may be community leaders with an interest in biomedical research. Reviewers are drawn from this panel and focus their reviews on the quality of the plan for stakeholder engagement. Second, we developed a scoring rubric, so we could include reviewers' results in the overall review process.

This chapter explores the engagement of community members in the Tufts CTSI peer review process. We describe the set of proposals that require stakeholder engagement plans, the key elements that must be included in a stakeholder engagement plan, methods for training researchers and reviewers about stakeholder engagement, and finally, the review process itself.

Proposals That Include Stakeholder Engagement Plans

Similar to most Clinical and Translational Science Awardees, Tufts CTSI sponsors pilot grant funding and graduate-level training in clinical translational science (CTS). Additionally, we support other funding mechanisms such as Community Health Catalyst grants. Each of these programs has a requirement for a stakeholder engagement plan for the proposed research. For example:

- The Pilot Studies Program seeks proposals with a focus on building interdisciplinary, multi-institutional research teams including investigators from the basic, clinical, and/or applied sciences.

- The CTS Graduate Program was the first MS/PhD program in clinical research in a biomedical graduate school and an academic medical center in the nation. It is designed for trainees who seek to translate research into improved clinical care and public health.
- Community Health Catalyst grants fund community-driven translational research projects by community-based organizations and investigators from Tufts CTSI partner organizations. The program aims to stimulate community-researcher partnerships that address pressing and overlooked health issues impacting the well-being of communities.

These programs are integral to Tufts CTSI's efforts to accelerate research and stimulate broadly engaged team science.

The Three Key Elements of a Stakeholder Engagement Plan

In 2018, Tufts CTSI began requiring a stakeholder engagement plan in submitted grant proposals for Pilot and Community Catalyst Awards and for graduate student thesis proposals required for a clinical translational science degree. The SCE Program team developed standards for the content of the plans based on a previously published guidance paper and tailored them to CTSI programs through dialogue and discussion among program directors and staff [1].

The goal of requiring stakeholder engagement plans is to promote inclusion of and accountability to stakeholders, and each one must describe which stakeholders to include and how they will be involved. Applications are expected to cover the following:

1. **Stakeholder identification, recruitment, and training.** Identify key stakeholders and develop specific plans for recruitment and training.
2. **Engagement in the research process.** How stakeholders will be (or were) involved in the planning, conduct, dissemination, and use of research.
3. **Dissemination of research results**. How the team will ensure that partner agencies and communities are included in plan for dissemination of research results.

Identification of Stakeholders Applicants are instructed to identify stakeholders guided by Concannon's 7Ps framework, which identifies key stakeholders to consider, including patients and the public, providers, purchasers, payers, policy makers, product makers, and principal investigators [2]. Proposals are expected to describe the rationale for including specific categories of stakeholders. Including key stakeholders early in the process improves the relevance of the research and the impact on public health by addressing questions of primary importance to each stakeholder.

Example: One thesis proposal outlined a sophisticated mathematical prediction tool for clinical decision-making. In developing this proposal, the student assessed currently available data, but did not include discussions with the clinicians involved in patient care.

The review panel flagged the failure to identify this key group of stakeholders and suggested that engagement of clinical decision-makers during the research design phase would improve the salience of the analysis. A mathematically rigorous model developed without stakeholder input was not sufficient to meet the thesis requirements.

The student rewrote their stakeholder engagement plan based on this feedback.

Students and applicants can find examples of relevant engagement techniques in the Tufts CTSI SCE Program webpage and in resources provided by the Pilot Studies Program. For community-based participatory research and patient-centered outcomes research, identification of stakeholders is an integral part of the research protocol. However, identification of stakeholders may be more complicated for earlier stage translational research, which generally uses advanced biomedical techniques to better understand disease mechanisms. These early-stage studies typically do not involve human subjects and require familiarity with the model systems used. Nonetheless, these studies can benefit from engagement with industry representatives or other stakeholders with insight into applications of early-stage discoveries.

Stakeholder Engagement Once identified, engaging specific individual stakeholders requires thoughtful planning. In stakeholder engagement plans, applicants must specify outreach approaches to be used or describe those that have already been initiated. There must be clear expectations for how stakeholders will be involved and communicate with the research team. In most cases, the budget will need to include resources for compensating stakeholders.

Tufts CTSI's network and resources may be helpful at this phase. The website for the SCE Program offers publications, web resources, and informational videos. In addition, the SCE Program and Tufts CTSI's Integrating Underrepresented Populations in Research (IUPR) Program offer expertise that can be accessed by investigators during consultation. For instance, investigators can access the expertise of Tufts CTSI's Stakeholder Expert Panel and consult with experienced researchers about methods for stakeholder and community engagement. These experts can also facilitate relationships with potential stakeholder groups.

The precise nature of stakeholder involvement will depend on the goals of the study, translational research phase, and other study specifics. Some studies may require fully cooperative partnered research; others may require more focused consultation during each phase of the project. Stakeholders may be engaged in defining the research question, outcome measures, and improving the design of the research protocol, or they may be involved in reviewing inclusion and exclusion criteria, ensuring they are clear and free of bias. In certain instances, people who have participated in prior trials may be most helpful by focusing on the research participant experience, to minimize unnecessary burden. Finally, many groups of stakeholders (e.g., patients with a rare chronic disease) may be able to assist the research team with participant recruitment strategies and later activities such as data analysis as appropriate.

Dissemination of Outcomes Generally speaking, stakeholders can assist with plans to ensure that the outcomes will be disseminated to the broader community of interest. Per Institutional Review Board (IRB) requirements, research participants are routinely informed of the progress and results of the study. It is important to distinguish that, while participants may be informed, the broader stakeholder community may be left out. When community-based organizations have assisted with study recruitment, they also expect to hear about the results of the research. While some funding sources may require community-wide dissemination of results, it is not a universalregulatory requirement, and community members often report feeling abandoned following completion of a study. This problem is exacerbated by the long timeline for academic results reporting. Typical dissemination plans for study results focus on presentations at scientific meetings and publications in peer-reviewed journals, but those are not necessarily available to the broader community and can use technical language that is not broadly accessible. While important for the progress of science, additional efforts to reach those more directly involved in the studies also promote the development of institutional relationships that make it easier to demonstrate the value of the research enterprise and engage community organizations in future research activities.

The stakeholder engagement plan, therefore, must contain an overview that will be the logical product of the study itself, stakeholder involvement, and the broader implications of the completed work. Tufts CTSI can help investigators allay their concerns about intellectual property and the need to avoid public discussion prior to peer-reviewed publication. There are a variety of community-based approaches for dissemination, including community meetings, local media or newspapers, and town hall-type forums.

Training and Support for the Preparation of Stakeholder Engagement Plans

The development of detailed stakeholder engagement plans is a complex undertaking that is relatively new to most clinical investigators. As a result, there is a need to provide clear guidance regarding exactly how to incorporate stakeholder engagement planning into translational research projects. We prepared training materials for investigators and graduate students who are developing stakeholder engagement plans, and these instructions are now available in a variety of different formats—as documents online, via webinars, and through in-person consultations. Over the 2 years since this process began, we have developed materials that explain the components of a stakeholder engagement plan, provide examples of exemplary prior submissions, and describe the review process and scoring criteria in detail.

After the first cycle during which pilot grants were subject to this new procedure, we conducted a review of the new Tufts CTSI stakeholder engagement process, including feedback from applicants. This was part of an ongoing evaluation of the stakeholder engagement requirements in the Pilot Studies Program. While results are preliminary, we are learning that many research investigators had not received prior training in stakeholder engagement.

To address these concerns, we produced the Tufts CTSI Pilot Studies Program Stakeholder Engagement Plan Toolkit. Developed by the pilot grant award project manager, the toolkit includes a series of case studies across the translation spectrum. It is made available to applicants as a resource for them during the application process. In addition to these materials, CTSI offers individual consultations, online and print resources, and question-and-answer format office hours for applicants to get help with their stakeholder engagement plans. Applicants are also referred to other relevant CTSI services. In additions, applicants can attend webinars and office hours for general guidance, and they can make appointments with the program manager for assistance specific to their applications.

Recruiting and Training Reviewers

To provide feedback on stakeholder engagement plans, we enlisted members of Tufts CTSI's Stakeholder Expert Panel. The Stakeholder Expert Panel is a roughly 25-member group of former patients, current and former research participants, community members, and community-based organizational representatives. Panel members are compensated for their time spent on projects and in meetings. The group members involved are motivated to support this process and many state that they feel it is important to be involved in this work as a way to improve the research process. This separate review ensured that stakeholder engagement plans were a meaningful component of the proposals and were considered in the evaluation of the overall assessment of each proposal.

Stakeholder-reviewers ranged from individuals familiar with the process of review through their involvement in patient-centered outcomes research to community activists with little training in research processes and methods. To ensure quality review, we trained stakeholder reviewers in two distinct sessions. The first session, delivered in-person or online, focused on both general issues related to clinical research and detailed descriptions of the grant review process. Participants were offered either a live webinar or review of online materials. The second session

Pilot Studies Program
Stakeholder Expert Panel Review

APPLICATION INFORMATION
Application ID:
Principal Investigator's Name and Affiliation:
Reviewer's Name:

STAKEHOLDERS	SCORE
Ability to identify key stakeholder groups and determine the role they play or may play in the proposed research project.	
RELEVANCE	SCORE
Ability to demonstrate explicit relevance of the project and its outcomes to the identified stakeholder groups and the public.	
APPROACH	SCORE
Rigor of the proposed stakeholder engagement plan to meet the proposed objectives and goals.	
OVERALL IMPACT	SCORE
Strengths	
Weaknesses	
Prompting questions (if any):	
Additional comments and/or suggestions (if any):	

Fig. 23.1 Scoring rubric for stakeholder engagement

training focused on the importance of the peer review process and the mechanics of review. Stakeholder-reviewers were introduced to the NIH (0 to 9) scoring system and oriented to the stakeholder engagement scoring rubric and worksheet (Fig. 23.1).

The second session consisted of meetings either in person or livestreamed with the leaders of the participating programs. In the case of pilot projects, this meeting was held with the scientific director of the pilot project program. For the student thesis proposals, reviewers were oriented by leadership from the clinical translational science graduate program.

Scoring Rubric

A scoring rubric was developed to provide a summary score from 0 to 9, mirroring the standard National Institutes of Health (NIH) rubric and score results. Points can be assigned in each of the three components: identification of stakeholder groups (as measured by depth of stakeholder relationship), ability to demonstrate relevance of proposed project outcomes to identified stakeholders, and rigor of proposed plans for stakeholder inclusion in developing research procedures and dissemination of outcomes. Reviewers are asked to assign each element a score in the range of one (top score) to nine. The committee comments and overall impact scores were then summarized and shared with the Scientific Review Committee for their consideration in overall scoring of the entire application.

Review Process and Integration into Overall Proposal Assessment

Once applications were received, they were distributed for review to stakeholder panelists. Each proposal was assigned at least two reviewers, and they were asked to complete the worksheets and submit them to CTSI staff. Once all reviews were submitted, an in-person review committee was held. Each application was presented by the primary reviewer, with additional discussion by a secondary reviewer. The entire panel was asked to reach agreement on a score from 0 to 9.

For our internal CTSI grants program, stakeholder engagement plan reviews were woven into the existing internal peer review process. The results of each review were presented to the overall scientific reviewer committee at the time that the applications were considered. In the case of pilot studies, the co-director of the committee stakeholder engagement component presented the comments and scores when scientific reviewers presented their reviews to the committee. Committee members considered the stakeholder panel review, along with the scientific reviews, in assigning priority scores for each application. Stakeholder reviewers were also welcomed to attend the review committee meetings and offer any additional input.

For graduate program thesis proposals, results of the review were presented to the program's Scientific Advisory Committee, which must approve each thesis proposal and completed thesis. The difference between Pilot and Community Health Catalyst proposal reviews, which were numeric, and the qualitative thesis reviews was best summarized by one reviewer who described their approach:

" … comments should be supportive and validating, while things that are identified as a weakness could help them fine tune their proposal. If [a student] read something and thought, 'Interesting, I never thought of it that way,' then that could be a positive thing."

In some cases, the committee asked the student to rewrite or resubmit the thesis proposal incorporating the comments from the stakeholder panel. Following the completion of the review, the authors of each proposal received written feedback from the stakeholder reviewer for their consideration. We also offered an opportunity for feedback concerning the stakeholder review in which students could ask additional questions or seek clarification on the recommendations they received. In addition, CTSI staff collated comments from the review committee, together with the previously submitted reviewer comments, and the evaluation worksheet for each submission.

Feedback on the Reviewing Process and Areas for Continued Exploration

To date, our stakeholder panel has reviewed more than 50 proposals. As we continue to carry out this process, we look forward to having a deeper understanding of the perceptions of stakeholder engagement among the grant awardees and trainees Tufts CTSI supports. During the first cycle of pilot reviews, we implemented a brief evaluation for the reviewers to complete. Based on this feedback we were able to determine which components were effective and which may need improvement. All agreed with the statements included in the evaluation and some offered suggestions to change the scoring, which was adjusted for Year 2 to make it more user friendly (Fig. 23.2).

Based on Year 1 feedback, we also provided more direct guidance on how much time to spend on each proposal and emphasized that while reviewers should read the whole proposal for context, their primary focus should be on the stakeholder engagement sections. One of our reviewers commended our iterative process. "The rubric was initially challenging... However, the rubric has been improved via a process of simplification and standardization," they said.

Going forward, we can rely on a series of resources that have been developed for stakeholder review of submissions to Tufts CTSI. These include detailed instructions for applicants and reviewers, PowerPoint presentations and agendas from in-person or live streamed meetings, and instruments for feedback from program chairs, proposers, and members of the stakeholder review committee.

At least two areas for continued exploration have been identified. To date, we have been reviewing only T2, T3, and T4 applications. However, a large number of proposals are early in the translation spectrum. Together with the active research exploration of the meaning of broadly engaged team science in these more basic research projects, we will be exploring developing specialized stakeholder engagement panels that will allow meaningful review of T0.5 and T1 applications. We also

Feedback on reviewing process	Strongly disagree	Somewhat disagree	Neither agree nor disagree	Somewhat agree	Strongly agree
The scoring rubric was clear and easy to follow	☐	☐	☐	☐	☐
The training on how to conduct a proposal review was well organized.	☐	☐	☐	☐	☐
The written guidance on how to conduct a proposal review was clear and understandable	☐	☐	☐	☐	☐
Communication about the process was prompt and my questions were answered	☐	☐	☐	☐	☐
I would recommend this to others	☐	☐	☐	☐	☐

Fig. 23.2 Feedback survey for stakeholder reviewers

recognize that inclusion of the stakeholder engagement plan in a proposal does not ensure its implementation. Future work will be needed to monitor the implementation of the stakeholder engagement plans in CTSI funded research.

References

1. Concannon TW, Grant S, Welch V, Petkovic J, Selby J, Crowe S, Synnot A, Greer-Smith R, Mayo-Wilson E, Tambor E, Tugwell P, Multi Stakeholder Engagement C (2019) Practical guidance for involving stakeholders in health research. J Gen Intern Med 34(3):458–463. https://doi.org/10.1007/s11606-018-4738-6
2. Concannon TW, Meissner P, Grunbaum JA, McElwee N, Guise JM, Santa J, Conway PH, Daudelin D, Morrato EH, Leslie LK (2012) A new taxonomy for stakeholder engagement in patient-centered outcomes research. J Gen Intern Med 27(8):985–991. https://doi.org/10.1007/s11606-012-2037-1

Chapter 24
Role of Broadly Engaged Team Science in the Inclusion of Minority Populations as Research Participants and in All Roles on Research Teams

Pamela B. Davis and Harry P. Selker

Abstract In the United States (US), racial disparities in health, health care, and medical research are striking. Although the contributors to health inequity are long-standing, systemic and beyond the scope of direct medical care, the health care enterprise has a responsibility to address those issues specific to its purview. These encompass the lack of proportionate representation of minorities among health professionals, the skew of research toward the majority population so that there is less evidence on which to base therapeutic decisions for minorities, and a lack of research and treatment relating to the social, economic, and environmental determinants of health. In this chapter, we address the two key needs for including minority populations in all aspects of clinical research and clinical trials. First, minority groups must be included among study participants in order for research to apply to these groups. Second, to generate relevant and well-designed research, there also must be representative diversity across all roles on research teams.

Keywords Broadly engaged team science · Inclusion of minority patients · Racial disparities in health · Therapeutic decisions for minorities

In the United States (US), racial disparities in health, health care, and medical research are striking. These disparities are completely unacceptable for a nation with the best trained physician and health workforce, the largest biomedical research enterprise, and the greatest wealth of all nations. Although the contributors to health

P. B. Davis
Case Western Reserve University, Cleveland, OH, USA

H. P. Selker (✉)
Tufts Clinical and Translational Science Institute, Tufts University, Boston, MA, USA

Institute for Clinical Research and Health Policy Studies, Tufts Medical Center, Boston, MA, USA
e-mail: hselker@tuftsmedicalcenter.org

© The Author(s), under exclusive license to Springer Nature Switzerland AG 2022

D. Lerner et al. (eds.), *Broadly Engaged Team Science in Clinical and Translational Research*, https://doi.org/10.1007/978-3-030-83028-1_24

inequity are longstanding, systemic and beyond the scope of direct medical care, the health care enterprise has a responsibility to address those issues specific to its purview. These encompass the lack of proportionate representation of minorities among health professionals, the skew of research toward the majority population so that there is less evidence on which to base therapeutic decisions for minorities, and a lack of research and treatment relating to the social, economic, and environmental determinants of health.

Among the many important efforts underway to address the disparities in health care, here we address the two key needs for including minority populations in all aspects of clinical research and clinical trials:

- First, minority groups must be included among study participants in order for research to apply to these groups.
- Second, to generate relevant and well-designed research, there also must be representative diversity across all roles on research teams.

Inclusion of Patients from Minority Populations in Clinical Research

Inclusion of minority patients in clinical research is critical. Studies have shown that specific racial/ethnic minority populations can have divergent disease courses and responses to treatment when compared with white populations. For example, African-Americans benefit most from a different progression of anti-hypertensive therapies than other patients, which affects treatment recommendations and ultimate health outcomes [1]. Additionally, mutations in colon cancers from African-American patients differ from those most common in other patients, suggesting that alternative therapeutic approaches might be necessary [2]. To detect differences in treatment needs among diverse populations requires inclusion of minority participants in sufficient numbers to allow for robust conclusions. This goal has been achieved in several recent trials, such as SPRINT or ALLHAT, but many trials in other clinical areas, such as in cancer, fall short [3, 4].

There is no single approach to assure inclusion of minority patients in trials, but a foundational requirement would be that the funders of clinical trials set the expectation for inclusion of minority participants and then provide appropriate resources for recruitment. Other recommendations include assuring that the research team itself is diverse, so that at least some members of the team are also members of the minority community. Community participants are reassured when at least some members of the team look like them. Establishing long-term relationships with members of the minority community, such as clergy, political leaders, and business leaders, can build trust and form alliances that facilitate participation in research. In addition, meeting potential participants in the community, as opposed to the academic health center, may also be important.

Two recommendations to improve minority participation in research emerge from these considerations. First, the funding agencies of research must require and support the recruitment of an appropriate mix of participants. Second, drawing on the collective wisdom of successful clinical research leaders, a compendium of advice for clinical research investigators who are intent upon inclusion of patients from minority populations in their research could be helpful.

Improving Diversity Across All Roles on Research Teams

Beyond the recruitment of minority individuals as study participants, to generate relevant and well-designed research, there must be diversity across all roles on research teams. The concept of broadly engaged team science is helpful for addressing this need [5]. This concept emphasizes that all stakeholders should be full members in the research team and involved in planning, executing, analyzing, and communication about the research.

This strategy sharpens the focus of research on those topics of most interest to the community. It also improves the practical execution of research because it is built on a foundation of assessment and understanding of its relevance to, and feasibility in, the population at hand. Moreover, for patients and community members, it can demystify the research process, increase trust, and increase confidence in and the adoption of research results. Many social scientists have long asked community members to review and improve their study protocols, disseminate results, and to build trust. This approach often requires years of engagement with the community before trust is established, and it often requires working physically in the community rather than always in academic buildings. It can challenge long-held assumptions and reveal flaws in prior research or plans. Reinforcing the importance of having patients involved in every step in the planning, execution, and dissemination of research, the Patient Centered Outcomes Research Institute (PCORI) was a leader in intentionally requiring the inclusion of representatives of patient populations on the research team, a foundational component of broadly engaged team science.

However, broadly engaged team science can be difficult to manage for academic researchers and may not fit conveniently into the operational models of academic health centers. The inclusion of non-experts on the team often requires a much greater investment of time, tact, and energy than working with a hand-picked team with considerable expertise. Projects may move more slowly if trust must be built at the outset, the needs of community members satisfied, and community members persuaded of the appropriate methodology. This longer timeline may be incompatible with the original plans, the grant period and funding, or the tenure clock. But in serving society's needs, larger health-related questions are difficult to answer without the cooperation and the concurrence of the community, since we now understand that socioeconomic factors play a major role in individual and community health.

In order to encourage and enhance broadly engaged team science, funders targeting clinical and translational research should be aware of the challenges to its appropriate execution in order to provide support for surmounting these challenges. Projects that provide flexible timelines and funding targeted at engaging the community even before the research begins may be especially useful. Modest pilot funding for such engagement would allow research groups to establish themselves in the community prior to launching larger projects. It would be important for granting programs that support infrastructure for patient-based research, such as Clinical and Translational Science Awards, to include long-term community engagement in their portfolio. Additionally, academic institutions must recognize the time and effort required to conduct this important research, which may have long lead times with little early apparent output, but then become very productive. Careful mentoring to maintain productivity and focus is important, and sufficient academic time and stable support personnel are crucial.

A broad collaborative effort among the stakeholders, including funders, institutions sponsoring research, investigators, and the community will be necessarily to address both the need for minority participation in studies and diverse representation among research team members. A variety of approaches are outlined above, but the specific mechanisms by which the goals are achieved may need to be tailored to the study at hand, or to the population that it is important to engage. Fundamental to all such improvements, however, is a background of trust and mutual respect among the stakeholders. Positive examples, such as the results of clinical trials with high minority enrollment (e.g., SPRINT and ALLHAT) and PCORI studies on the engagement of all stakeholders at all stages, should be celebrated and widely reported. These success stories also illustrate the importance of conducting research with minority participants so that the resulting data can be more broadly applicable to real-world populations. For example, ALLHAT demonstrated that the order of addition of antihypertensive drugs to a regimen for control of the blood pressure is best done differently for Black and White populations. This realization may encourage leading funders to post more effective mandates for inclusion of minorities as research participants. At the same time, the institutional hosts for such research should review their expectations and requirements for success of individual faculty members and their teams, to allow for the additional time and resources required to engage all appropriate team members in the planning and conduct of the research. As the funding agencies increasingly require such inclusive strategies, the academic health centers must rise to meet them.

References

1. Taylor AL, Wright JT Jr (2005) Should ethnicity serve as the basis for clinical trial design? Importance of race/ethnicity in clinical trials: lessons from the African-American Heart Failure Trial (A-HeFT), the African-American Study of Kidney Disease and Hypertension (AASK), and the Antihypertensive and Lipid-Lowering Treatment to Prevent Heart Attack

Trial (ALLHAT). Circulation 112(23):3654–3660; discussion 3666. https://doi.org/10.1161/circulationaha.105.540443

2. Guda K, Veigl ML, Varadan V, Nosrati A, Ravi L, Lutterbaugh J, Beard L, Willson JK, Sedwick WD, Wang ZJ, Molyneaux N, Miron A, Adams MD, Elston RC, Markowitz SD, Willis JE (2015) Novel recurrently mutated genes in African American colon cancers. Proc Natl Acad Sci U S A 112(4):1149–1154

3. Group SR, Wright JT Jr, Williamson JD, Whelton PK, Snyder JK, Sink KM, Rocco MV, Reboussin DM, Rahman M, Oparil S, Lewis CE, Kimmel PL, Johnson KC, Goff DC Jr, Fine LJ, Cutler JA, Cushman WC, Cheung AK, Ambrosius WT (2015) A Randomized Trial of Intensive versus Standard Blood-Pressure Control. N Engl J Med 373(22):2103–2116. https://doi.org/10.1056/NEJMoa1511939

4. Wright JT Jr, Dunn JK, Cutler JA, Davis BR, Cushman WC, Ford CE, Haywood LJ, Leenen FH, Margolis KL, Papademetriou V, Probstfield JL, Whelton PK, Habib GB (2005) Outcomes in hypertensive black and nonblack patients treated with chlorthalidone, amlodipine, and lisinopril. Jama 293(13):1595–1608. https://doi.org/10.1001/jama.293.13.1595

5. Selker HP, Wilkins CH (2017) From community engagement, to community-engaged research, to broadly engaged team science. J Clin Transl Sci 1(1):5–6. https://doi.org/10.1017/cts.2017.1

Chapter 25
Rewarding Team Science in Tenure and Promotion Practices: An Operational Imperative for the Academic Research Enterprise of the Twenty-First Century

Augusta Rohrbach and Caroline Attardo Genco

Abstract To succeed in a research-intensive academic environment, the team science approach must be embraced by faculty not only in preparing trainees for the workforce as part of the educational mission of the university, but also in advancing scholarship throughout the research spectrum from basic to translational science research. Tenure and Promotion Guidelines traditionally uphold a standard of inquiry that reflects the core principles of academic excellence, as represented by publications, extramural funding, and other accepted impact factors; however, how faculty are acknowledged and rewarded for team science has not been adequately addressed due to the historical significance of the single investigator model of research productivity despite the prevalence of, and necessity for a team science approach. This chapter will focus on how this problem is manifested and potential solutions that focus on alignment of Tenure and Promotion guidelines with team science core principles to optimize outputs of research and scholarship.

Keywords Collaborative research · Tufts Springboard · Tenure and promotion guidelines

A major challenge facing the academic research enterprise is how to sustain and grow a robust, diverse workforce in a climate where breaking traditional norms around the evaluation of research and scholarship is often met with resistance. Most will agree that there is a pressing need to address complex, multilayered scientific

Supplementary Information The online version of this chapter (https://doi.org/10.1007/978-3-030-83028-1_25) contains supplementary material, which is available to authorized users.

A. Rohrbach · C. A. Genco (✉)
Tufts University, Boston, MA, USA
e-mail: Caroline.Genco@tufts.edu

© The Author(s), under exclusive license to Springer Nature Switzerland AG 2022
D. Lerner et al. (eds.), *Broadly Engaged Team Science in Clinical and Translational Research*, https://doi.org/10.1007/978-3-030-83028-1_25

231

problems in a nuanced and sophisticated way that is best achieved by a team science approach. Furthermore, studies have shown that diverse teams that bring a variety of perspectives based on lived experience achieve optimal results, informed by cutting-edge methods, and enhanced by approaches to problem solving from multiple and different perspectives [1].[1] Thus a team science approach aligns with the research imperative to do the very best science, but it also clears a path to take into consideration background, age, gender, sexual orientation, race, ethnicity, culture, religion, geography, disability, socioeconomic status, area of expertise, level of experience, thinking style, and skill set within the context of a research agenda, bringing scientific inquiry into contact with the social, political, and economic contexts that shape the world we live in and produce world-class scientific results.

To succeed in a research-intensive academic environment, the team science approach must be embraced by faculty not only in preparing trainees for the workforce as part of the educational mission of the university, but also in advancing scholarship throughout the research spectrum from basic to translational science research. Tenure and promotion guidelines traditionally uphold a standard of inquiry that reflects the core principles of academic excellence, as represented by publications, extramural funding, and other accepted impact factors; however, how faculty are acknowledged and rewarded for team science has not been adequately addressed due to the historical significance of the single investigator model of research productivity despite the prevalence of, and necessity for a team science approach [2, 3]. This chapter will focus on how this problem is manifested and potential solutions that focus on alignment of Tenure and Promotion guidelines with team science core principles to optimize outputs of research and scholarship.

Incentivizing the Team Science Model to Invigorate Research and Scholarship

Most academics would agree that we no longer need to make a case for the value of collaboration in research and scholarship. Indeed, ample evidence exists that collaboration fosters innovation [4].[2] For decades, countless articles, chapters, and volumes bear out the importance of collaboration to scientific discovery [5–7]. From the perspective of the funding agencies, both federal and private, collaboration across disciplines has also become one of the prerequisites to succeed in an

---

[1] "Overwhelming evidence suggests that teams that include different kinds of thinkers outperform homogeneous groups on complex tasks, including improved problem solving, increased innovation, and more-accurate predictions—all of which lead to better performance and results when a diverse team is tasked to approach a given problem" [1].

[2] "Convincing evidence (Wuchty et al. 2007) shows that coauthored research, as compared to single-researcher work, more often leads to high knowledge impacts as well as to commercial uses of research as reflected in patents. Further, the success of collaborative teams attracts more collaborators, thus accelerating the growth of research teams (Parker and Hackett 2012)" [4].

increasingly complex and competitive research landscape. Indeed, many funding opportunities not only expect a research *team*, but require a track record of successful collaboration to present a plausible case for the impact on today's multi-layered research challenges that grantors seek to address.

Like many other research-intensive universities, Tufts University has invested significantly in incentivizing the team science model to invigorate research and scholarship. In 2011, under the leadership of President Anthony Monaco and Provost David K. Harris, Tufts University launched Tufts Collaborates. The program was structured to encourage the essential first steps in interdisciplinary collaboration by supporting new pilot projects that engage at least two disciplines and cross school lines. The goal of this program was to establish collaborative research efforts that would likely result in competitive research proposals to federal and foundation granting agencies. In operation for a decade, the program spawned numerous cross-school collaborations with the goal of promoting a culture of collaboration and producing increased extramural funding.

With a collaborative culture firmly embedded, Tufts Collaborates was retired and replaced by Tufts Springboard in 2020. As part of Vice Provost for Research Caroline Attardo Genco's strategic vision to increase large scale, multifactorial research impacts, the objective of this program is to stimulate high-impact collaborative research that will lead to a competitive extramural funding proposal, such as an R01 or the equivalent, and with eventual externally funded programmatic funding for centers of excellence. Springboard builds on the team science approach that Tufts Collaborates cultivated. However, a key innovation of this new program is to provide a range of administrative support with the understanding that the managerial aspects of large-scale team science approaches require more than just financial resources to succeed. In addition, the program has also sought to advance the University's Antiracism Initiatives based on its 2021 Institutional Audit and Targeted Action Plan while also recognizing the latest research that shows the importance of diversity on research teams to catalyze innovative thinking and research outcomes, placing an emphasis on diverse teams and work that addresses structural inequities across the research spectrum [8, 9].[3]

In addition to seed funding programs, in January 2017, Tufts University launched a more sustained endeavor to support team science through an institutional Research and Scholarship Strategic Plan (RSSP) to promote future innovations in Research and Scholarship (R&S) at the university [10]. The RSSP process identified key areas in which Tufts should invest and that addressed large-scale issues using interdisciplinary approaches. Determining thematic priorities was a multi-stage process that included 95 one-on-one interviews, 16 focus groups, and a university-wide survey—a process that took place over the course of 18 months. This work identified five broad areas from which faculty leaders in these priority areas formed long-term research goals. These efforts culminated in the establishment of faculty-led

---

[3] AlSheblie, Rahwan, and Woon found that increased diversity with regard to ethnicity, age, gender, and affiliation was associated with increased 5-year citation count, with ethnic diversity having the greatest impact [9].

Priority Research Clusters (PRCs) built around existing areas of excellence, to expand opportunities for cross-disciplinary collaboration, and to do this with a view toward the greatest potential for future innovations and global impact.

Value of Team Science Approach

As a university-wide, long-term investment, the Priority Research Clusters are supported by the Office for the Vice Provost and their events, pilot funding, and other recruitment efforts are advertised across a range of university channels. This increased visibility helps attract junior, mid-career, and senior faculty from across the university. The PRCs were charged with the goal to increase their faculty members and have succeeded in consistently engaging faculty from all eleven schools and centers in addition to researchers from Tufts Clinical and Translational Institute (CTSI), Tufts Medical Center, Tufts University School of Medicine's primary teaching hospital, and Wellforce, TMC's parent health system. By design, they utilize a team science approach—bringing together a diverse collection of faculty united in their interest to solve complex, multifaceted research problems. PRCs create a sense of belonging focused on a common mission, especially important to faculty engaged in interdisciplinary research that does not fit well into departmental silos. Thus, the PRCs are also an ideal locus to create the conditions for inclusive excellence and fit well with the University's Antiracism Initiatives based on its 2021 Institutional Audit and Targeted Action Plan [8]. Tufts is now implementing evidence-based and innovative approaches to create a just, equitable, and inclusive research, teaching, and service environment in the university and the PRCs are an important landing pad for such efforts. These clusters sponsor opportunities to receive recognition through seed funding, internal and external research seminars, workshops and retreats, and as avenues for dissemination of research results. To foster these efforts and reap the benefits of a team science approach, Tufts University provides funds and also offers ongoing administrative support to enable the development of a cohesive team empowered by a shared vision for success.

The PRCs describe outcomes of shared success in an annual report presented to the Vice Provost for Research and senior leadership. These include: 1) Faculty satisfaction, hires and retention; 2) Funding to support ongoing research; 3) Visibility of work nationally/internationally with recognition from target audiences; 4) High impact publications related to the priority research cluster; and 5) Opportunities for training students and other trainees. As outlined in these five shared measures of success, PRC activities provide multiple forms and sources of mentoring, research-related activities, and support a thriving intellectual community while also improving research outcomes. PRCs provide a structured network of mentors designed to encourage and support early career faculty as their teams pursue innovative research outcomes that exceed the dimensions of single discipline solutions. These include training by senior faculty mentors, and providing peer-to-peer and near-peer mentoring. The PRCs represent Tufts team science approach: nesting individual mentoring and sponsor relationships tailored to individual goals and needs within cluster mentoring to support collaboration, diversity, team science, and inclusion into existing priority research cluster communities. While these mentoring activities are definitely accounted for in the tenure and promotion processes, further work may be needed for a more uniform understanding that such activities are highly valued, especially from the faculty. Indeed, what the PRC experience suggests is that mentoring, while typically considered as part of faculty service, may more rightly be thought of in the team science context as an important part not only of the research process but also a form of the research product. The recommendation here would be to invite faculty to count mentoring, when in the team science context, as a research indicator.

PRCs also develop an awareness as to the importance of stewardship. For instance, leveraging institutional funds is critical to the group's success and long-term sustainability, highlighting the need to operate according to a responsible plan to promote success beyond the immediate term. Balancing research activities and infrastructure development is one of the challenges of PRC leadership that the RSSP process has surfaced and for which its members actively work to identify effective solutions. RSSP seed funding is used by all PRCs to support their activities, ranging from conferences, chalk talks, course releases, seed grants, and workshop/development for publications on the PRC theme. While the stewardship of these activities are taken into account in the tenure and promotion processes, we recommend that further action may be needed to emphasize the value and importance of the curatorial work that large scale collaboration requires.

In addition to the standard measures of productivity, mentoring and stewardship demonstrate progress toward the common goal of charting a path forward for Tufts University as an innovative, civically engaged, student-centered, tier-one research university. Collectively, each PRC serves to advance Tufts' educational mission, expand its research expenditures, and raise its research profile. In acknowledgement of what it takes to become, remain, and advance as a collective, collaborative research team, it is important to include mentoring and stewardship as elements of productivity in tenure and promotion review. Likewise acknowledgement of these important activities in attracting and retaining a dynamic and diverse faculty must be a priority for Tufts University.

Clearly, the PRCs have the power to shift the culture of academic science to one of collaboration, community, and belonging. In supporting the PRCs, Tufts University affirms that team science demands a unique set of skills that are not covered in textbooks. To be successful, team members must, in addition to performing cutting-edge science, also hone the ability to appreciate, synthesize and operationalize the diversity of approaches, viewpoints, and training with a focus on the research goal. Leaders of successful project groups require what Bozeman and Youtie call "the social and managerial aspects of research teams and the factors affecting research collaboration" [4]. Leaders of teams manifest the very same personal and professional qualities that are markers of good mentors, but with a focus on the research mission and finding ways to ensure that each and every team member contributes fully. Early career faculty engaged in team science have access to mid- and senior level faculty who offer them hands-on experience and professional development opportunities promoting self-efficacy, an important characteristic for long-term productivity and career satisfaction.

Furthermore, the PRCs capacity to create the conditions for inclusive excellence through mentoring and stewardship have recently figured prominently in the University's efforts to "find and eradicate any structural racism at Tufts and to take the steps necessary to become what every member of our community would view as an anti-racist institution" [11]. The deep engagement and training of mentors and mentees within this cluster model will help shift the culture of academic science to one of collaboration, community, and belonging to improve the outcomes of a diverse cohort of early career faculty. The PRC structure offers Tufts University a measurable context for improvement of support and equitable evaluation of collaborative, influential research and scholarship. Creating a space for mentoring and stewardship as indicators of research productivity provides an important corollary to assigning value to work supporting diversity, inclusion, equity, and justice (DEIJ), more broadly speaking. Rewarding DEIJ work and related activities that build and sustain a culture of inclusion are essential for a thriving twenty-first century research enterprise [1].

Role of Team Science in Tenure and Promotion

Despite the robust set of resources available to encourage team science, from internal seed fund programs to large extramural grants, the measures of productivity have not necessarily been understood uniformly in assigning appropriate credit to faculty engaged in team research. Tufts' tenure and promotion processes have some mechanisms in place for evaluating the performance of cohort members in multi-investigator collaboration, including: (1) The Provost's requirement that deans' letters on promotion and tenure candidates include comments on the candidates' interdisciplinary research collaborations to solve complex problems, including collaborations between STEM and non-STEM fields (including the humanities); (2) Consistent advising from department chairs, mentors, and academic deans throughout the pre-tenure period to make contributions to collaborative projects clear, both in reviews for the second and fourth year reviews, as well as in the tenure and promotion application; and (3) Letters from collaborators for the tenure file. Candidates for tenure are encouraged to solicit "Additional Letters" from collaborators, which provide information to the tenure and promotion committee and the Tufts administration about the role of different investigators in a collaborative project, paper, or grant. Certainly, projects on which a tenure/promotion candidate is an intellectual leader and/or central part of a collaboration are given credence similar to individual projects, and *all* collaborative projects are accounted for in the evaluation process and thoroughly discussed at promotion and tenure meetings. However, these policies and processes are not necessarily understood by those impacted, including the faculty themselves. Thus, an additional recommendation is to educate and further communicate with faculty, trainees, and administrators alike.

Understanding the nature of team science begins with acknowledging the functional similarities between research performed by a single-investigator and work conducted by a team. In both cases, the value of the work is measured by its impact. However, there are significant operational differences that multiply as research moves from a single-investigator model to a team science approach (Fig. 25.1). An integrated research team requires an added set of activities that reach beyond its research specific activities which include frequent meetings, regulating processes, establishing team norms around expectations, intellectual property, scientific attribution, and authorship. While the term "team science" may better reflect all these activities than "research collaboration," it should not exclude the complex research collaborations between the sciences, the humanities, and the arts that are often needed to address complex problems and are so valuable at a comprehensive university like Tufts. Indeed, teams that bring the STEM fields into contact with the arts, humanities, and social sciences require as much, if not more, careful stewardship and mentoring to flourish and achieve their goals.

Multifactorial, twenty-first century problems require carefully coordinated team approaches shaped by consistently implemented organizational practice. To this end, tenure and promotion guidelines can help teams create and adhere to clear expectations for sharing credit and authorship, routinizing best practices in the field through the University's most powerful reward—tenure and promotion—by recognizing these steps as part of the research process, as essential as presentations and grant applications are in laying the groundwork for long-term success. For instance, Tufts, like many other institutions, has implemented a policy that defines authorship attribution and thus provides guidance to collaborators according to four criteria:

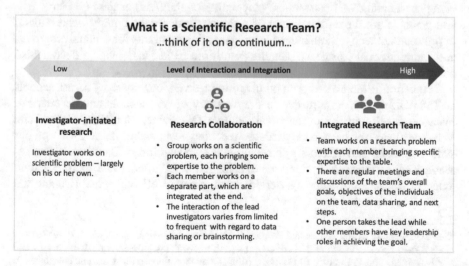

Fig. 25.1 What is a scientific research team? The degree of interactions and the need for integration increases as the number of investigators increases [4]

1. Contributing substantially to the conception or design of the study or to the acquisition, analysis or interpretation of data for the study;
2. Drafting the manuscript submitted for publication or revising it critically, if needed, for important intellectual content.
3. Approving the final version that will be published; and
4. Agreeing to be publicly accountable for the accuracy or integrity of the publication's conclusions and the supporting research.

These four principles align closely with standards in use to identify intellectual contribution in a team science context. The criteria is being institutionalized by the recommendation that candidates be careful to document their individual contributions to collaboration as outlined in the Tenure and Promotion Guidelines [12].[4] Many teams begin their collaborative relationships by setting forth roles and responsibilities as well as other expectations in a research agreement. Such documents can, in turn, be submitted as part of the tenure dossier. At present, Tufts is instituting new guidelines that will not only make this path clearer to all stakeholders—from candidate to mentors, department chairs, tenure committees, deans, and outside experts invited to review materials.

The research enterprise is evolving to recognize the importance of team science and thus aligning tenure and promotion policies with team science approaches will reflect the requirements investigators face in a competitive funding environment. The trend among funding agencies is to sponsor grants with multiple PIs as well as large grants to fund centers, programs, and international collaboration. Ideally, policies should encourage what, indeed, are considered the best practices of many fields and disciplines to create the conditions for innovative research with broad and lasting effects. As with publication trends, funded grants, sponsored by federal and non-federal sources alike are frequently spread across multiple institutions. Thus, being "first author" or "last author" (depending on the field) or the PI on large federal grants is not the only indicator of research productivity, quality, achievement, or professional recognition. Indeed, many large federal grants for centers, programs, and international projects require multiple PIs and well documented collaborations.

Interestingly, tenure and promotion guidelines vary considerably across schools at Tufts University, in part, due to the diversity of our schools and centers. For instance, faculty in the professional schools (Medicine, Nutrition, Dental, and Veterinary) do not have undergraduate teaching responsibilities and two of our schools (Dental and Veterinary) have clinical responsibilities. Thus, while there is recognition of the classic "three- or four-legged stool" model that requires excellence in scholarship, teaching, service, and possibly clinical work (Dental and

---

[4] See Statement 12 of the Tenure and Promotion Guidelines, *Evidence of scholarly contributions distinct from those of mentors and collaborators*. In many fields collaboration is necessary and highly valued, and the ability to establish fruitful collaborations with excellent colleagues is viewed positively. Nonetheless it is essential that the candidate's individual contributions be clearly explained and demonstrated [12].

Veterinary) as metrics for tenure or advancement, variability is inherent in the definition of excellence in all three/four areas according to each school's needs/standards and each school has its own policy. This system is inherently adaptable to crediting measurable aspects of team science if a solid rubric for performance in teams is available. Collaborative science can be further evaluated through the inclusion of collaborators as professional references to be included in the tenure file [12].[5][6] As a supplement to defined contributions within an authorship policy, such supporting letters from collaborators can be used to clarify levels of contribution to a team science project and its research outcomes. As these examples illustrate, promotion and tenure-relevant evaluation of a faculty member's contributions to team science projects is possible given a carefully crafted set of definitions and measurement tools, coupled with training in their use by those charged with shepherding candidates through the process.

Next Steps for Supporting Team Science

Tufts presents a strong record of supporting, recognizing, and celebrating collaborative work of diverse teams, which often yields the most transformative and influential research outcomes. While differences among school guidelines in a research-intensive university setting need to be recognized, the universal evaluation and acknowledgment of the nature and function of team science as a major accelerator of the research mission that is taking place could be further enhanced and communicated. Tufts University has underwritten the team science model of collaboration and transdisciplinary approaches through a series of important programs for over a

---

[5] See "Procedures for Deciding the Award of Tenure Candidates" [12]: For tenure must submit the following materials to the ATP at the time that the Dean of Academic Affairs writes the ATP Committee to initiate the tenure review:

- A current (within the last year) CV;
- A letter requesting consideration for tenure;
- A personal statement describing the candidate's research and teaching goals and accomplishments, focusing on accomplishments during the entire tenure-track appointment;
- Copies of five to ten recent published articles, reports, or other appropriate works of which the candidate is sole author or an author who has made a major substantive contribution, representative of his/her work;
- A list of six to twelve suggested professional references. Most of these should be persons holding tenured or similar senior level academic appointments. The list should include the names and contact information for former students, mentors and other collaborators, as well as recognized leaders in the candidate's field who have not been associated with the candidate. For lateral hires, references received as part of the search may be counted among the references for consideration for tenure; and
- A teaching portfolio demonstrating effectiveness of courses, mentorship and other instructional activity, with a complete list of past and present Academic and Thesis Advisees and graduate trainees.

[6] There was no mention of collaboration as a consideration in the Dental School documents.

decade, namely, Tufts Collaborates, Springboard, and the Priority Research Clusters (PRCs) established by the Institutional Research and Scholarship Strategic Plan (RSSP) as well as seed funding opportunities supported by the cooperative efforts between Tufts University and our clinical partners at Tufts Medical Center [13–15]. The next steps needed to continue the upward trend created by the University's support of team science efforts in key signature seed funding programs include:

1. Further communicate the value of team science to the faculty and ensure that such efforts are accounted for in promotion and tenure processes.
2. Continue the progress that has been recently achieved at Tufts by requiring that deans' letters on promotion and tenure candidates include comments on both individual research and collaborative research addressing complex problems.
3. Consider the mentoring and stewardship required by team science efforts as both important and valuable research processes as well as research products.
4. Craft a set of definitions and measurement tools, coupled with training in their use by those charged with shepherding candidates through the process.

Finally, the proposed policy reforms in faculty evaluation and academic advancement processes discussed here, and already articulated in the Tufts plan to become an anti-racist institution, will move the university toward the inclusive excellence for all faculty and is critical to its mission as a student-centered research university dedicated to the creation and application of knowledge. Tufts is committed to providing transformative experiences for students and faculty in an inclusive and collaborative environment where creative scholars generate bold ideas, innovate in the face of complex challenges, and distinguish themselves as active citizens of the world [16].

References

1. Swartz TH, Palermo AS, Masur SK, Aberg JA (2019) The science and value of diversity: closing the gaps in our understanding of inclusion and diversity. J Infect Dis 220(220 Suppl 2):S33–S41. https://doi.org/10.1093/infdis/jiz174
2. Klein JT (2008) Evaluation of interdisciplinary and transdisciplinary research: a literature review. Am J Prev Med 35(2 Suppl):S116–S123. https://doi.org/10.1016/j.amepre.2008.05.010
3. Klein JT, Falk-Krzesinski HJ (2017) Interdisciplinary and collaborative work: framing promotion and tenure practices and policies. Res Policy 46(6):1055–1061. https://doi.org/10.1016/j.respol.2017.03.001
4. Bozeman B (2017) The strength in numbers: the new science of team science. Princeton University Press, Princeton
5. Katz JS, Martin BR (1997) What is research collaboration? Res Policy 26(1):1–18. https://doi.org/10.1016/S0048-7333(96)00917-1
6. Beaver DD (2001) Reflections on scientific collaboration (and its study): past, present, and future. Scientometrics 52(3):365–377. https://doi.org/10.1023/A:1014254214337
7. Bozeman B, Boardman C (2014) Research collaboration and team science: a state-of-the-art review and agenda. Springer International Publishing AG, Cham
8. Institutional audit and targeted actions workstream: final report Tufts as an Anti-Racist Institution (2021). Tufts University

9. AlShebli BK, Rahwan T, Woon WL (2018) The preeminence of ethnic diversity in scientific collaboration. Nat Commun 9(1):5163. https://doi.org/10.1038/s41467-018-07634-8
10. A brighter world through research and scholarship (2018) Tufts University strategic plan for research and scholarship. Tufts University
11. Tufts as an Anti-Racist Institution: Executive Summary (2021). Tufts University
12. Tufts University Arts, Sciences, and Engineering Faculty Handbook 2021 (2021) Tufts University
13. Tufts Collaborates (2020) https://provost.tufts.edu/teaching-research/seed-grants-for-teaching-and-research/tufts-collaborates/. Accessed 18 May 2021
14. Research and Scholarship Strategic Plan (2021). https://viceprovost.tufts.edu/research-scholarship-strategic-plan. Accessed 18 May 2021
15. Internal Seed Funding Programs (2021). https://viceprovost.tufts.edu/internal-seed-funding-programs. Accessed 18 May 2021
16. Mission, vision & themes. https://www.tufts.edu/about/mission-vision. Accessed 2 Feb 2021

Epilogue

Debra Lerner, Thomas W. Concannon, and Marisha E. Palm

In 2017, Wilkins and Selker introduced broadly engaged team science, describing it as a potential pathway for clinical and translational research to have a greater and more sustained impact on the public's health [1]. The book is a starting point for defining this new framework in terms of a specific knowledge base and core set of team research practices. This collection of chapters explores broadly engaged team science from the perspectives of clinical and translational science researchers, academic administrators, clinicians, and community members. It is apparent from these chapters that broadly engaged team science is being applied to a vast terrain of research topics, questions, methods, and organizational arrangements all the while remaining grounded in the specific knowledge and reality of individuals and groups, who are key stakeholders.

Intersection of Broadly Engaged Team Science with Other Scientific Traditions

It would be an oversimplification to regard broadly engaged team science as simply a blending of team science and community and stakeholder engagement, which could be achieved by adding stakeholders to research teams but not changing team

D. Lerner
Tufts Clinical and Translational Research Institute; Institute for Clinical Research and Health Policy Studies, Tufts Medical Center, Boston, MA, USA

T. W. Concannon
RAND Corporation, Boston, MA, USA

Tufts Clinical and Translational Science Institute, Boston, MA, USA

M. E. Palm
Tufts Clinical and Translational Research Institute; Institute for Clinical Research and Health Policy Studies, Boston, MA, USA
e-mail: dlerner@tuftsmedicalcenter.org

© Tufts Medical Center, RAND Corporation 2022
D. Lerner et al. (eds.), *Broadly Engaged Team Science in Clinical and Translational Research*, https://doi.org/10.1007/978-3-030-83028-1

dynamics or culture. In this book, broadly engaged team science is re-imagined as a distinct scientific approach that is substantive, complex and purpose-driven, that draws upon three strands of scientific thought: a science in society perspective, team science, and community and stakeholder engaged research.

A science in society perspective, drawing from Kuhn, regards the work of scientists as *influenced by* the social and historical context and, in turn, *influencing of* these contexts [2]. Arguably, the emerging interest in broadly engaged team science can be viewed as partly the result of the nation's health and health care challenges, most recently the pandemic, an increased awareness of health disparities and systemic barriers to equity and inclusion, and demands for greater accountability from the public and private sector institutions that are in a position to effect change in the public's health.

The mutual, bi-directional influences of science and society are always present but in many instances have been ignored in the work of scientists, many of whom may wish to control such influences in the name of objectivity. Broadly engaged team science embraces the idea that such influences are essential; they should be made explicit in research and intentionally given voice. This perspective is likely to be more comfortable for some clinical and translational scientists than for others and better aligned with some phases of research than others. Presumably, some of the scientists who focus on patient care and health policy issues may find it easier to acknowledge the influence of social and political forces on their research questions, procedures, and research products, while others from the biomedical sciences may not. Similarly, scientists involved in later translational stages of research may be more willing to forge new research partnerships in order to achieve meaningful change in health. It remains to be seen whether broadly engaged team science will become the norm among a wider range of scientists across the entire translational spectrum.

Broadly engaged team science also has roots in team science, recognizing that new discovery is often best translated to clinical applications and care only after multiple scientific disciplines have contributed insights. Medical science grew quickly in the twentieth century, resulting in increasing specialization of disciplines before it became apparent in the twenty-first century that complex and multi-faceted problems require a multidisciplinary, collaborative approach. In 2003, the National Institute of Health (NIH) set out a roadmap to move biomedical research away from single discipline, single principal investigator silos and towards encouraging multidisciplinary work with investigators working together as a team [3]. In the years since the NIH Roadmap, the NIH CTSA Program has taken up the goal of team science, hosting a team science training workshop in 2009 and identifying team science as a critical element of clinical and translational research [4].

Team science has proliferated in the last two decades, with researchers beginning to study the science of team science. In 2015, the National Academy of Science published a report that identified gaps in the evidence base, such as the effectiveness of programs to prepare and support team science and evaluation of the processes and outcomes of team science [5]. Team science has developed useful lessons for cross-disciplinary working and multi-investigator research; however, the work continues to be inwardly focused on scientists or researchers, often remaining closed off to other types of expertise. Moving towards broader engagement in team science opens the door to wider stakeholder input and teamwork.

Broadly engaged team science is also rooted in community and stakeholder engaged research, which originated in the 1960s and gained further momentum after the Institute of Medicine 'Quality Chasm' report in 2001 [6]. That report and subsequent studies showed the presumed link between established scientific evidence and real-world patient care practices was broken. At that time, clinical care guidelines—built on the painstaking accumulation and synthesis of evidence—were being used correctly about 50% of the time in US clinical settings [7].

Extensive legislative, policy, and program research reforms followed, most of which included new requirements for community and stakeholder engagement in federally funded research [3, 8–11]. The Patient-Centered Outcomes Research Institute (PCORI), established in 2010, set out to advance the development and use of rubrics, frameworks, and reporting guidelines to bring engagement work into the science mainstream [10]. As a result of these and other initiatives, the number of publications focused on this area has grown exponentially over the past two decades, and there are now journals that focus specifically on engagement, with public members acting as co-editors and reviewers. Much of the thinking that has already been done about flattening hierarchy, sharing power, and building both openness and trust will inform broadly engaged team science. Principles that support equity and transparency, and practices that create room for co-learning and development, will be important foundations from which to broaden team inclusivity and perspective.

Transformation

A recurrent theme of this book is that for clinical and translational science to be truly transformational it must start by transforming itself. The preceding chapters describe transformations occurring in many different ways and across an array of clinical disciplines including neonatology, nephrology, oncology, genetics, pharmaceutical and device development, pediatrics, nutrition, infectious disease, obstetrics, environmental health, and orthopedics. The authors share examples of broadly engaged team science perspectives across the translational spectrum, from as early as the inception of research questions through organizational processes and finally to the dissemination and implementation phases of research findings. Often, the early, pre-study phase of research included detailed consideration of the downstream goals and challenges of sustainability. The authors also document innovations at the scientific team level that include ground-breaking collaborations between clinical and translational scientists and social movements, law enforcement, engineering students, patients and patient advocates, care navigators, and multiple community-based organizations and community coalitions of historically marginalized racial, ethnic, and cultural groups, particularly in the neighborhoods of Boston and surrounding areas.

The experiences described in these chapters emphasize the critical importance of building trust in research and improving access to research resources and financial supports—in effect, sharing a larger slice of the research dollars pie. In many instances, this involves innovating with resources, tools, and frameworks, including changing communication dynamics and patterns that perpetuate distance and distrust between scientists and others. In addition, it is clear that we need innovative approaches for advancing knowledge of the processes by which community coalitions influence the sustainability of new health care interventions, as well as new process improvement techniques to enhance team effectiveness.

How can academic departments and institutions move to adapt in ways that encourage, rather than conflict with, the goals of broadly engaged team science? At Tufts Medical Center, changes are underway to provide material and operational support to research team members who are outside the traditional academic enterprise. Across CTSAs, changes are underway to recognize engagement work as a promotion criterion for research faculty.

These and the other, many changes that can be seen across the research ecosystem may not be implemented without challenge. Adaptations in some cases have the potential to change deeply entrenched academic systems. Broadly engaged team science will require both structural and cultural changes. The preceding chapters highlight changes that were beginning to occur in research teams, research infrastructure, training and education, processes for eliciting and reviewing proposals for sponsored research, grant and contract development and administration, and in academic hiring, promotion and tenure committees.

Looking Ahead

The convergence of several forces including the pandemic, lingering disparities in health and health care, and renewed focus on social and economic injustices addressed by the Black Lives Matter movement and others are stark reminders of the existence of science skepticism and mistrust. Segregating science activities has had the unintended consequence of fueling the fires of mistrust and in some cases failing to respond to our most pressing health needs. This book is a first step towards building a knowledge base and set of practices to support new collaborations built upon a perspective of clinical and translational science as a collective endeavor and authentic collaboration between research scientists and stakeholders.

References

1. Selker HP, Wilkins CH (2017) From community engagement, to community-engaged research, to broadly engaged team science. J Clin Transl Sci 1(1):5–6. https://doi.org/10.1017/cts.2017.1
2. Kuhn T (1962) The structure of scientific revolutions. International Encyclopedia of Unified Science, vol II. The University of Chicago

3. Zerhouni E (2003) Medicine. The NIH roadmap. Science 302(5642):63–72. https://doi.org/10.1126/science.1091867
4. Institute of Medicine (2013) The CTSA Program at NIH: Opportunities for Advancing Clinical and Translational Research. The National Academies Press (US), Washington, DC. https://doi.org/10.17226/18323.
5. Cooke N, Hilton ML (2015) Enhancing the effectiveness of team science. The National Academies Press, Washington, DC. National Research Council (2015) Enhancing the Effectiveness of Team Science. The National Academies Press (US) Washington, DC. https://doi.org/10.17226/19007.
6. Institute of Medicine Committee on Quality of Health Care in A (2001) Crossing the quality chasm: a new health system for the 21st century. National Academies Press (US) Copyright 2001 by the National Academy of Sciences, Washington, DC. https://doi.org/10.17226/10027
7. McGlynn EA, Asch SM, Adams J, Keesey J, Hicks J, DeCristofaro A, Kerr EA (2003) The quality of health care delivered to adults in the United States. N Engl J Med 348(26):2635–2645. https://doi.org/10.1056/NEJMsa022615
8. Medicare Prescription Drug, Improvement, and Modernization Act of 2003 (2003)
9. The Patient Protection and Affordable Care Act (2010)
10. Spurring Community Involvement in Research (2021) https://www.pcori.org/engagement
11. NIH National Center for Advancing Translational Sciences (2021) https://ncats.nih.gov/ctsa/about

Index

© Tufts Medical Center, RAND Corporation 2022
D. Lerner et al. (eds.), *Broadly Engaged Team Science in Clinical and
Translational Research*, https://doi.org/10.1007/978-3-030-83028-1

Printed in the United States
by Baker & Taylor Publisher Services